Self-Assessment Colour Review of

Thoracic Imaging

SJ Copley MD, MRCP, FRCR
Consultant Radiologist and Honorary Clinical Lecturer,
Hammersmith Hospital,
London, UK

DM Hansell MD, FRCP, FRCR
Professor of Thoracic Imaging,
Royal Brompton Hospital,
London, UK

NL Müller MD, PhD, FRCPC
Professor of Radiology,
Vancouver General Hospital,
Vancouver, Canada

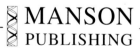

MANSON
PUBLISHING

Classification of cases

Cases may appear under more than one category; references are to case numbers

airway disorders 2, 5, 29, 60, 73, 86, 89
anatomical abnormalities 67, 94
cardiogenic disorders 46
diaphragmatic disorders 41
diffuse parenchymal disease 10, 16, 17, 18, 30, 36, 39, 48, 65, 74, 75, 78, 81, 83, 88, 96, 98
hereditary and congenital disorders 13, 20, 29, 31, 50, 58, 70, 76, 94, 95
imaging modalities 9, 37, 59
immune-mediated disorders 2, 5, 8, 30, 74, 89
infective diseases (non-tuberculous) 12, 27, 35, 49, 63, 68, 90
mediastinal lesions 15, 23, 32, 42, 47, 61, 64, 71, 72, 77, 82, 95, 99

multi-system disorders 2, 8, 10, 48, 61, 71, 74, 75, 81
occupational/environmental disease 3, 16, 55, 79, 88, 92, 97, 98
paediatrics 27, 50, 70, 73, 87
pleural and chest wall disease 3, 7, 12, 14, 24, 55, 57, 79
post-surgical complications 14, 43, 56, 59, 89
tuberculosis 1, 38, 52, 84, 85, 93
tumours, benign/non-pulmonary 6, 23, 47, 53, 62, 82
tumours, malignant/pulmonary 4, 9, 15, 22, 25, 28, 32, 33, 37, 42, 44, 51, 55, 72, 80, 83, 91, 100
vascular disorders 19, 26, 45, 58, 59, 69, 77, 94

Copyright © 2005 Manson Publishing Ltd
ISBN: 1–84076–062–1

A CIP catalogue record for this book is available from the British Library.

For full details of all Manson Publishing Ltd titles please write to:
Manson Publishing Ltd, 73 Corringham Road, London NW11 7DL, UK.
Tel: +44(0)20 8905 5150
Fax: +44(0)20 8201 9233
Email: manson@mansonpublishing.com
Website: www.mansonpublishing.com

Commissioning editor: Peter Altman
Project manager: Paul Bennett
Page layout: Initial Typesetting Services
Colour reproduction by Tenon & Polert Scanning Ltd, Hong Kong
Printed (in China) by New Era Printing Company Ltd, Hong Kong

Preface

Thoracic imaging plays a part in the assessment of patients in a wide variety of disciplines, not just respiratory medicine. The chest radiograph is a ubiquitous first-line investigation in many acutely ill patients, and the accurate interpretation of such a relatively humble technique still remains a challenge. The radiographic findings may guide further more sophisticated imaging techniques such as computed tomography (CT). Advances in CT such as high-resolution CT (HRCT) have led to increased sensitivity for the detection of pulmonary disease and increased specificity for diagnosis. Helical or spiral CT allows for much faster scanning times, multiplanar reconstructions, and optimization of intravenous contrast enhancement. Hence CT pulmonary angiography is now the first-line radiological investigation in many cases of suspected pulmonary embolus, allowing direct visualization of thrombus, even down to the level of the subsegmental arteries.

Advances in nuclear medicine, such as positron emission tomography (PET) and CT/PET, have had a large impact on the assessment and staging of many neoplasms, especially lung cancer. The role of magnetic resonance imaging (MRI) remains limited but it can be useful for the assessment of some thoracic neoplasms.

This book is primarily aimed at medical students and physicians and surgeons with an interest in thoracic imaging; the cases included in this book vary from very simple to more demanding and esoteric cases that will challenge even experienced radiologists. Thus in some cases the diagnosis is straightforward, while others are more complicated and designed to demonstrate the intricacies of the more sophisticated techniques such as HRCT and, hopefully, encourage further reading. Radiologists in training will also find the book useful as a self-assessment exercise before specialist examinations.

Abbreviations

AAT alpha-1-antitrypsin
ABPA allergic bronchopulmonary aspergillosis
ACE angiotensin-converting enzyme
ACTH adrenocorticotrophic hormone
AIDS acquired immune deficiency syndrome
AP anteroposterior projection
ARDS acute respiratory distress syndrome
(c)ANCA (cytoplasmic) antineutrophil cytoplasmic autoantibodies
AVM arteriovenous malformation
BAC bronchioloalveolar cell carcinoma
BOOP bronchiolitis obliterans organizing pneumonia
CCAM congential cystic adenomatoid malformation
CD4 surface antigen on helper T lymphocytes
CF cystic fibrosis
CLE congenital lobar emphysema
CMV cytomegalovirus
COP cryptogenic organizing pneumonia
COPD chronic obstructive pulmonary disease
CRP C-reactive protein
CT computed tomography
CTPA computed tomography pulmonary angiogram
DAD diffuse alveolar damage
DL_{CO}/TL_{CO} total diffusion coefficient for carbon monoxide
ET endotracheal
ECG electrocardiogram
ESR erythrocyte sedimentation rate
FDG fluorodeoxyglucose
FEV_1 forced expiratory volume in 1 second
FVC forced vital capacity
HIV human immunodeficiency virus

HPOA hypertrophic pulmonary osteoarthropathy
HRCT high-resolution computed tomography
IgE immunoglobulin E
IPF idiopathic pulmonary fibrosis
JVP jugular venous pulsation
K_{CO} adjusted gas transfer coefficient
KS Kaposi's sarcoma
LAM lymphangioleiomyomatosis
MAA macroaggregated human serum albumin
MAI *Mycobacterium avium intracellulare*
MRI magnetic resonance imaging
NTM nontuberculous mycobacteria
pCO_2 partial pressure of carbon dioxide
PA posteroanterior projection (chest radiography)
PAS periodic acid Schiff stain
PCP *Pneumocystis carinii* pneumonia
PET positron emission tomography
PIOPED prospective investigation of pulmonary embolism diagnosis
PLCH pulmonary Langerhan's cell histiocytosis
PMF progressive massive fibrosis
RDS respiratory distress syndrome
RV residual volume
SVC superior vena cava
TB tuberculosis (*Mycobacterium tuberculosis*)
TLC total lung capacity
UIP usual interstitial pneumonia
VATS video-assisted thoracoscopic surgery
VA accessible alveolar volume
VC vital capacity
VQ ventilation-perfusion (scan)
VSD ventriculoseptal defect

Glossary of terms

Air-trapping: abnormal retention of air within the lung on expiration. It is seen on expiratory CT as areas showing a less than normal increase in attenuation.

Architectural distortion: abnormal displacement of pulmonary structures (bronchi, vessels, fissures) resulting in a distorted appearance of the lung anatomy. It is most frequently seen in fibrotic lung disease.

Bronchiectasis: irreversible bronchial dilatation which is localized or diffuse. Bronchial wall thickening and mucus impaction are often seen in both large and small airways.

Centrilobular: a structure (bronchiole or artery) or disease process which involves the centre of the secondary pulmonary lobule.

Consolidation: an increase in lung opacity, demonstrated on radiographs or CT, that results in obscuration of underlying vessels or bronchial margins. It represents replacement of alveolar air by fluid, cells, or other material. It should be differentiated from ground-glass opacity (which is grey, rather than white) where there is no obscuration of bronchovascular margins, on CT.

Cyst: a thin-walled (<3 mm thick), well-defined air- or fluid-containing lesion. It normally refers to an air-filled lesion on HRCT.

Emphysema: permanent, abnormal enlargement of airspaces distal to the terminal bronchiole, with destruction of the alveolar walls (pathology definition). It is seen on HRCT as decreased attenuation areas of destruction, usually without visible walls.

Expiratory CT: HRCT scans performed during end-expiration to demonstrate air-trapping.

Ground-glass opacity/opacification: a hazy increase in lung density on HRCT which does not obscure the margins of bronchovascular structures. A nonspecific finding which can result from interstitial thickening or fibrosis, airspace filling, or a combination of both.

Helical (spiral) CT: the principle of helical or spiral CT involves continuous rotation of an X-ray beam and detectors around the patient while the table moves through the X-ray gantry to produce a volumetric data set. Any scan acquired on this modern type of scanner will be 'helical' or 'spiral'. The term is not synonymous with CT pulmonary angiography (CTPA).

HRCT: the principle of high-resolution computed tomography involves the use of very thin (1 mm) sections and a high spatial frequency algorithm to produce highly detailed images of the lung parenchyma.

Honeycombing: multiple, often adjacent cystic airspaces ranging in size from a few millimetres to several centimetres in diameter, bounded by clearly defined walls (which are often thick, reflecting the fibrous nature of the walls). Honeycombing usually results from, and is associated with, pulmonary fibrosis.

Interlobular septum and interlobular septal thickening: a connective tissue structure which marginates the edge of a secondary pulmonary lobule and contains veins and lymphatics. These septa measure about 0.1 mm in thickness and are not usually seen in healthy subjects. The septa can be abnormally thickened by fibrosis, oedema or cells, allowing them to be visualized (most conspicuous in the periphery of the lung). This sign is the equivalent of the radiographic Kerley 'B' line.

Interstitium: the fibrous supporting structure of the lung parenchyma.

Intralobular interstitium and intralobular interstitial thickening: the fine interstitial network within the secondary pulmonary lobule (excluding the interlobular septa). It is not normally visible on HRCT but when thickened results in a very fine reticular or 'net-like' appearance.

Mosaic perfusion: inhomogeneity of lung attenuation with the blacker areas of lung being abnormal, with vessels in these regions appearing of reduced calibre or attenuated. It is most common with airways disease, but may reflect vascular obstruction or abnormal ventilation.

Nodule: a small focal opacity of varying size, which may be well or poorly defined.

Opacification: indicates an increase in attenuation or density of the lung parenchyma (normal lung is nearly black) and includes consolidation (white lung) and ground-glass opacity (grey lung).

Peribronchovascular interstitium: the connective tissue which encloses the bronchi and hilar vessels and extends from the pulmonary hila into the lung periphery.

Peribronchovascular thickening: thickening of the peribronchovascular interstitium resulting in apparent thickening of the bronchial wall and increase in size of the pulmonary arteries. The thickening can be smooth or nodular.

Secondary pulmonary lobule: the smallest unit of lung marginated by connective tissue septa. The secondary pulmonary lobules are usually bounded by interlobular septa containing veins and lymphatics and are supplied by bronchioles and arteries which are within the centre of the structure. A single secondary pulmonary lobule is normally made up of a variable number of acini, is roughly polyhedral in shape, and measures 1–2.5 cm in diameter.

Terminal bronchiole: the last purely conducting airway that does not participate in gas exchange.

Traction bronchiectasis: bronchial dilatation and irregularity caused by surrounding retractile pulmonary fibrosis.

Tree-in-bud: filling of bronchioles by fluid, pus, or mucus, resembling a branching tree about to bud. It is usually seen in the lung periphery.

Window level and window width: each CT section is a matrix of three-dimensional elements (voxels) containing a measurement of X-ray attenuation, arbitrarily expressed as Hounsfield units (HU): water measures 0 HU, air -1000 HU (so that lung parenchyma is approximately -600 HU), fat -80 HU, soft tissue 40–80 HU, and bone 800 HU. In order to display images of such varying densities, appropriate window settings need to be used, depending on the density of interest. The window width determines the number of HU to be displayed, with any densities greater than the upper limit displayed as white and any below the limit as black. Between these two limits, the densities are displayed as different shades of grey. The median density is the window centre or level.

1 A 21-year-old male from Zambia presented with a fever, night sweats, and malaise. He had developed the symptoms several weeks before presentation. On examination, he was cachectic, but not clubbed and had a slight pyrexia (37.5°C; 99.5°F). He was not immmunocompromised (CD4 count was normal) and had a mild leucocytosis. His chest radiograph is shown (1).

What are the possible diagnoses?

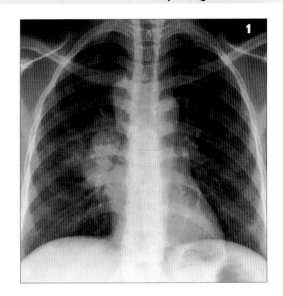

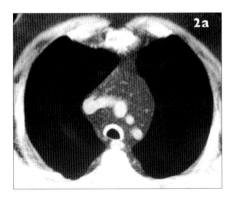

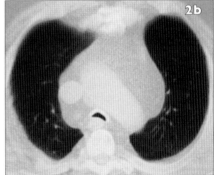

2 A 60-year-old male presented with dyspnoea, wheeze, and stridor several months previously. He had a history of intermittent painful swelling of his auricular cartilage. He had no other relevant past medical history. His blood tests were normal. Lung function tests showed an obstructive defect. The chest radiograph was normal. An inspiratory CT was performed (2a, viewed on soft tissue windows), supplemented with an end-expiratory image (2b, viewed on lung windows).

i. What is the abnormality?

ii. What is the likely diagnosis?

iii. What are the treatment options?

I, 2: Answers

1 The chest radiograph shows right paratracheal, right hilar lymphadenopathy and subcarinal nodes with loss of the upper azygo-oesophageal line (1). There is also subtle right mid-zone consolidation. The diagnosis was primary tuberculosis (TB). The radiological differential also includes lymphoma, metastatic disease (less likely in view of the patient's age), and sarcoidosis.

The radiographic features typical of primary TB include a focal pneumonia and lymphadenopathy in the adjacent lymph drainage pathway. The hilar lymphadenopathy is usually unilateral, with contiguous mediastinal node involvement. Lymphadenopathy may be more prominent in patients of African or Asian origin. The right lung is more commonly involved than the left, and lymph nodes may cause airway narrowing resulting in segmental or lobar atelectasis. Cavitation has been described in 10–30% of cases.

The radiographic features of pulmonary TB in patients with AIDS are influenced by the degree of immunosuppression. In patients with mild immunosuppression (depends on the CD4 count >0.2 × 10^9/l; 200/mm³), the features tend to be those of reactivation TB, including upper lobe consolidation, nodules, and cavitation. However, if the CD4 count is <0.2 × 10^9/l; 200/mm³, the features usually resemble primary TB, being characterized by the presence of lymphadenopathy with or without associated consolidation and lack of cavitation.

2 i. The CT images show abnormality of the trachea, which is thick-walled and calcified, with sparing of the posterior tracheal membrane (2a, b). On the end-expiratory images, there is tracheal collapse with the posterior membrane bowed anteriorly. Note the excessive mediastinal fat in this patient, who had been treated with corticosteroids for several months.

ii. The appearances are those of relapsing polychondritis, a rare disease of unknown aetiology characterized by recurrent inflammation of cartilage. Structures that are most often affected include the nasal cartilage, the pinna, and the cartilage-containing large airways. The disease is commonest in the fifth decade and there is an equal sex incidence. There is an association with other autoimmune diseases such as rheumatoid arthritis. Histopathological findings are chondral and perichondral inflammation with chondrolysis.

Respiratory tract involvement is a common and potentially life-threatening complication and may involve the large, cartilage-containing airways from the trachea to the segmental bronchi. The stenoses may be multiple, single, dynamic, or fixed and diffuse involvement may occur. The chest radiograph is often normal, although areas of atelectasis may be seen. CT demonstrates airway thickening, calcification, and collapse on end-expiration. Multiplanar reconstructions may be useful to guide treatment such as stenting.

iii. The treatment options include long-term steroids (as in this patient) to reduce airway inflammation, although more invasive techniques such as tracheostomy or airway stenting may be required.

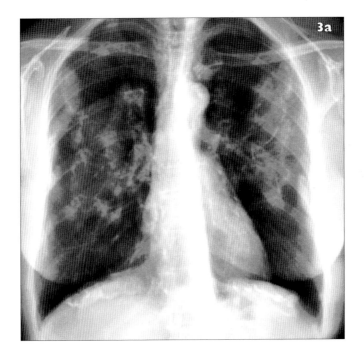

3 A 55-year-old female presented with a chronic nonproductive cough. She was anxious as her father had died of lung cancer caused by exposure to asbestos. He had worked as a packer in an asbestos factory. She had never smoked and did not keep any pets. She had had a total thyroidectomy in the past. The patient was well on examination with no abnormal physical signs. Serum biochemistry and full blood count were normal. Spirometric and plethysmographic lung function indices were normal.

i. What does the PA chest radiograph (3a) show?

ii. What is the likely cause?

3: Answer

3 i. The chest radiograph shows large, irregular, confluent opacities projected over both lungs and the diaphragmatic surface (3a). The opacities are partly calcified and resemble 'holly leaves' in outline. In some areas the opacities are well-defined, and in the right mid zone an opacity can be seen arising from the pleural surface with well demarcated edges. The bronchovascular markings can be seen clearly through the opacities seen 'en face' and no parenchymal distortion is present. The costophrenic angles are clearly defined. A CT shows

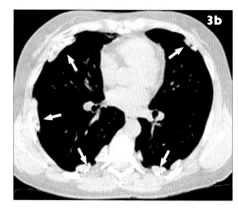

the calcified opacities to be arising from the pleural surface with well circumscribed edges (3b, arrows). No diffuse pleural thickening or parenchymal changes suggestive of asbestosis are seen. The radiographic and CT appearances are typical of benign pleural plaques due to asbestos exposure.

ii. Pleural plaques are the commonest manifestation of asbestos exposure, and bilateral scattered calcified pleural plaques can be regarded as virtually pathognomonic of asbestos exposure. Pleural plaques are uncommon in females, as most asbestos workers in the developed world are male. In this case, the patient's exposure occurred as a child when she helped her mother to wash her father's overalls at home. Pleural plaques are discrete elevated areas of hyaline fibrosis almost invariably arising from the parietal pleura. Despite much speculation, the pathogenesis of pleural plaques remains uncertain. It is now thought that short asbestos fibres reach the parietal pleura by passage through lymphatic channels, where they excite an inflammatory reaction, whereas the largest fibres, amphiboles, are retained in the lung parenchyma. Pleural plaques tend to lie adjacent to relatively rigid structures such as the ribs, vertebral column, and the tendinous portion of the diaphragm. According to radiographic studies, the characteristic sites are on the posterolateral chest wall between the seventh and tenth ribs, on the lateral wall between the sixth and ninth ribs, on the dome of the diaphragm, and the mediastinal pleura, particularly over the pericardium. This distribution is largely borne out by CT studies, although on CT plaques seem to be more profuse beneath the anterior aspects of the upper ribs (an area poorly demonstrated by standard radiographic views).

Pleural plaques slowly progress in size and amount of calcification with time, independent of any further exposure. Pleural plaques are not usually associated with impairment of lung function and there is no evidence that they undergo malignant degeneration into mesothelioma.

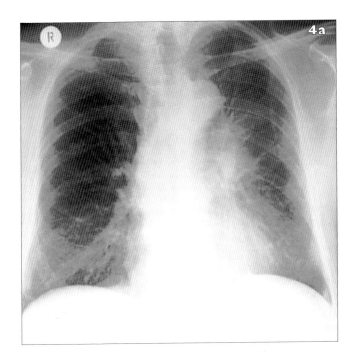

4 A 70-year-old male presented with a nonproductive cough but no episodes of haemoptysis. He was a retired council worker and smoked 20 cigarettes a day. On examination, he was plethoric and wheezy, but not clubbed or cyanosed. Decreased air entry was noted anteriorly over the left chest wall on auscultation, but no dullness to percussion. There were no abnormal findings in the cardiovascular or abdominal systems. Full blood count and urea and electrolytes were normal. The ESR was mildly elevated.

i. What does the PA chest radiograph show (4a)?

ii. What is the likely cause?

iii. What imaging investigation should be performed next?

4: Answer

4 i. The PA chest radiograph shows hazy increased density of the left hemithorax and obstruction of the left heart border (**4a**). The silhouette of the aortic knuckle is maintained. The left hemithorax is of slightly decreased volume, with a small juxtaphrenic diaphragmatic peak seen through the heart shadow. The trachea is also slightly deviated to the left. The left hilum is elevated, with the left main bronchus more horizontal than normal and the lower lobe bronchus more vertical. The appearances are those of a left upper lobe collapse, confirmed on the lateral chest radiograph (**4b**). Note that the major fissure is displaced anteriorly on the lateral radiograph and has a slight convexity superiorly (arrows). The radiographic features of a complete left upper lobe collapse are typical, although the aortic knuckle is classically obscured in cases with relatively mild volume loss. With more extensive volume loss, as in this case, the outline of the aortic knuckle is preserved as the hyperexpanded apical segment of the left lower lobe takes the place of the posterior segment of the upper lobe. The oblique fissure is usually concave on the lateral radiograph in a simple left upper lobe collapse and the slight convexity is suspicious of an underlying bronchial neoplasm.

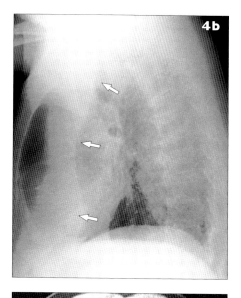

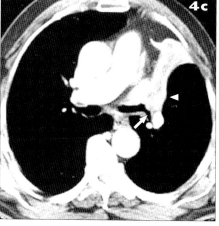

ii. The likely cause in an elderly smoker is a bronchogenic carcinoma obstructing the left upper lobe bronchus.

iii. The next imaging investigation of choice would be a contrast-enhanced CT. The CT shows the collapsed left upper lobe as a wedge-shaped density anteriorly (**4c**). There is a slight convexity posteriorly in the outline of the major fissure, suggestive of an underlying mass (arrowhead). An endobronchial lesion is demonstrated (arrow). The findings were confirmed at bronchoscopy and biopsy revealed a squamous cell carcinoma.

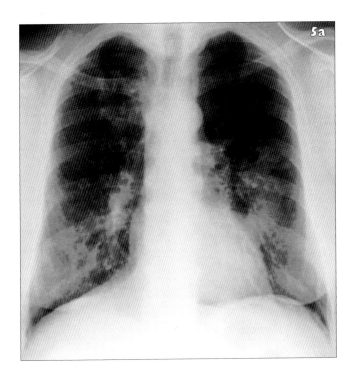

5 A 58-year-old female had been followed for 30 years for recurrent cough with yellow sputum and wheeze. She developed asthma and eczema at 4 years of age, which was initially worse during the summer with attacks of winter bronchiolitis. Her symptoms had gradually worsened from the age of 21 and currently she was breathless on minimal exertion with a productive cough and occasional pleuritic chest pain. She was cushingoid and mildly dyspnoiec at rest. On auscultation she had widespread wheezes. Lung function tests (predicted values) showed FEV_1: 47%; TLC: 121%; RV: 175%; K_{CO}: 78%. Sputum grew *Haemophilus influenzae*, with no fungal growth. The total IgE level was raised at 502 IU/ml (normal range 3–15 IU/ml), with a raised *Aspergillus fumigatus*-specific IgE level of 9.48 (range 0–0.35 kU/l). The CRP was high at 23 (normal range 0–10 mg/l) with a normal eosinophil count and negative precipitins to *Aspergillus*. Her chest radiograph is shown (5a).

i. What is the diagnosis?

ii. What are the major diagnostic criteria for this condition?

5: Answer

5 i. The chest radiograph shows normal volume lungs with perihilar peribronchial thickening and an area of opacification in the left midzone (**5a**). This has a rather lobulated appearance peripherally resembling a 'gloved finger', consistent with a bronchocele. The appearances are suggestive of allergic bronchopulmonary aspergillosis (ABPA). A subsequent HRCT after treatment demonstrated bronchiectasis in a predominantly proximal and central distribution (**5b, c**).

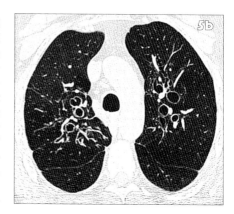

Aspergillus sp. is a ubiquitous dimorphic fungus which is present in soil and water. There are many species, but *A. fumigatus* is the most common pathogen in humans. It causes a wide spectrum of pulmonary disease, ranging from mycetoma formation in pre-existing chronic cavities in an immune-competent host to life-threatening invasive aspergillosis in the immunocompromised host. ABPA typically occurs in long-standing asthmatics, but is also frequent in patients with cystic fibrosis, and runs a relapsing and remitting course characterized by wheeze, dyspnoea, and cough. The fungus colonizes the airways, which contain abnormally thickened mucus, and

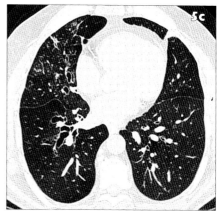

provokes both type 1 and type 3 immune reactions. The marked inflammatory response leads to bronchial plugging, bronchial damage, and bronchiectasis.

ii. The major criteria for diagnosis are: asthma; blood eosinophilia; immediate skin reaction to *Aspergillus* sp. antigens; raised IgE levels; pulmonary opacities; and central bronchiectasis. Minor criteria include *Aspergillus* sp. in the sputum and late skin reactivity.

Radiological changes are either acute and transient or chronic and permanent. Acute changes are characterized by consolidation which is often multifocal (80%), bronchocele formation (i.e. mucoid impaction seen as 'bunches of grapes' or 'gloved fingers'), and atelectasis of segments, lobes, or even an entire lung. Permanent changes are of proximal bronchiectasis and upper lobe fibrosis. The treatment of ABPA consists primarily of corticosteroids. Both chest radiographs and serum IgE levels are useful in monitoring disease activity and aggressive therapy may be needed to prevent the progression of ABPA.

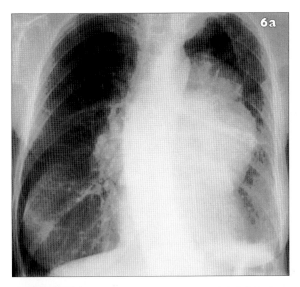

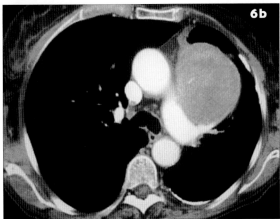

6 A 61-year-old female presented after having a routine chest radiograph prior to having a hysterectomy. She had been feeling nonspecifically unwell for a few months but had no other complaints. She had a history of tuberculous pleurisy in the past, many years previously. On examination, she was clubbed but there were no other abnormalities. Routine blood tests and pulmonary function tests were all normal. Her chest radiograph and CT are shown (6a, b).

Describe the radiological findings.

6: Answer

6 A large intrathoracic mass is demonstrated on the radiograph within the left hemithorax (6a). It obscures the left heart border. The left hilar structures can be seen projected through the abnormality. The aortic arch and descending aorta can still be seen. Pleural thickening is seen in the left hemi-thorax, especially at the apex. The CT shows a large mass of mixed contrast enhancement adjacent to the mediastinum on the left. It appears very closely opposed to the main pulmonary artery. There is a small 'tail' of soft tissue which is seen anteriorly and extends to the pleural surface (6c, arrow). There is calcified pleural thickening and volume loss within the left hemithorax consistent with previous TB empyema. The mass was resected and found to be a localized fibrous tumour of the pleura (previously known as pleural fibroma, fibrous mesothelioma, or benign mesothelioma).

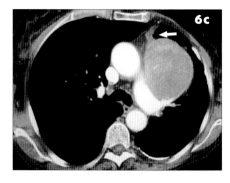

Histopathologically, localized fibrous tumours consist of spindle cells separated by collagen. The term 'benign mesothelioma' is a misnomer as these tumours are not mesotheliomas and may have a spectrum from benign lesions to malignancy. There is no association with asbestos exposure, although a link with previous radiotherapy has been reported. Most arise from the visceral pleura, with a smaller number arising from the parietal pleura. The lesions are often pedunculated. The tumours often grow very slowly and patients are often asymptomatic, the abnormality sometimes being found incidentally on chest radiography. Some patients have hypertrophic pulmonary osteoarthropathy and clubbing and, if the tumour is very large, hypoglycaemia may be a presenting feature. There is an equal sex incidence and patients between the ages of 45 and 65 years are usually affected.

On chest radiography, a large mass (up to 30 cm in diameter) is often seen and it is sometimes difficult to identify a pleural origin due to the large size (as in this case). If small, sometimes an obtuse angle at contact with the pleura can give a clue that the lesion is pleural in nature, although presence of the pedicle may result in an acute angle of contact. Another feature (which can also be appreciated on CT) is a change in position of the lesion depending on the orientation of the patient, again due to the presence of a vascular pedicle. The mass often demonstrates decreased attenuation centrally on CT due to necrosis, and heterogeneous enhancement with intravenous contrast enhancement. A small number calcify, but there are no specific features that allow accurate distinction of benign from malignant lesions (apart from local invasion in malignancy) and the lesions are often resected to allow histopathological evaluation of the entire lesion.

7 A 24-year-old female presented with recurrent right-sided pleuritic chest pains over 1 year. She reported the symptoms at the same time as menstruation. On examination, she was well, not in respiratory distress. Her full blood count and urea and electrolytes were normal.

i. What are the two subtle abnormalities on the chest radiograph (7a)?

ii. What is the likely diagnosis?

iii. What further investigations may be helpful?

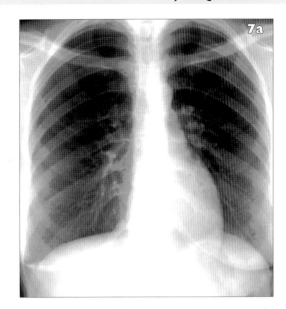

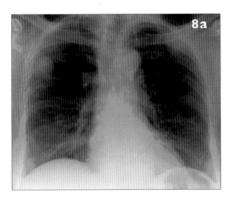

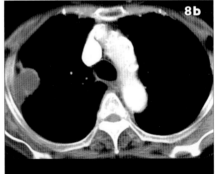

8 A 62-year-old female presented with a few weeks' history of lethargy and night sweats. She had a long history of seropositive rheumatoid arthritis and was on methotrexate. On examination she was apyrexial, with deformity of both her hands (ulnar deviation and joint swelling) consistent with her known erosive arthropathy. Subcutaneous nodules were also found at the extensor surfaces of the elbows bilaterally. As part of her investigations, a chest radiograph and CT were performed (8a, b).

i. What is shown?

ii. What is the possible diagnosis?

7, 8: Answers

7 i. The chest radiograph shows a very subtle right pneumothorax. The lung edge is shown by the arrows (7b). There is loss of the right costophrenic angle caused by a small pleural effusion at the right base. The upper margin of the pleural fluid shows a very straight line instead of the normal curved meniscus seen in a straightforward pleural effusion, indicating the presence of air within the pleural space (hydropneumothorax). This sign is another clue to the pneumothorax, which is easy to miss on the radiograph.

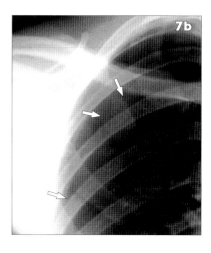

ii. The suspected diagnosis was a catamenial pneumothorax due to endometriosis. Pleuro-diaphragmatic endometriosis is a rare cause of a spontaneous pneumo- and haemothorax. Typically, small self-resolving pneumothoraces recur at the time of menstruation. The vast majority are right-sided (nearly 90%). The pathogenesis is controversial, but is thought to be due to a combination of diaphragmatic defects and diaphragmatic and pleural endometriotic implants.

iii. The pleural effusion was tapped under ultrasound guidance and was found to be heavily bloodstained, consistent with a haemothorax. The patient subsequently had pelvic MRI which revealed an endometriotic cyst in her left ovary. Laparoscopy revealed multiple peritoneal endometriotic implants.

8 i. The radiograph shows bilateral, well-defined nodules in the upper zones (8a). The CT shows one of the lesions peripherally in the right upper lobe with slightly lower attenuation than the muscles of the chest, which is suggestive of necrosis (8b).

ii. The diagnosis (confirmed by percutaneous needle biopsy of the lesion in the right upper lobe) was of necrobiotic rheumatoid nodules.

Histopathologically, pulmonary rheumatoid nodules are identical to subcutaneous rheumatoid nodules and are characterized by a necrotic centre surrounded by palisading histiocytes, plasma cells, and lymphocytes. There may also be adjacent non-necrotizing vasculitis. The majority of patients have coexisting subcutaneous nodules and long-standing rheumatoid arthritis although, in some cases, the nodules may pre-date the joint disease by several years. Pulmonary nodules are a relatively unusual manifestation of rheumatoid lung disease, and are commoner in males. Radiologically, they are well defined, sometimes multiple, vary in size, and have an upper, mid-zone, and peripheral predilection. They cavitate in about one-half of cases. Nodules may increase in size and number, resolve spontaneously, or wax and wane with the activity of the joint disease and subcutaneous nodules. Often they are radiologically indistinguishable from malignant lesions and histological confirmation is required.

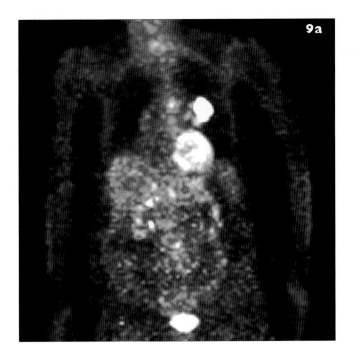

9 A 65-year-old female smoker presented with cough and haemoptysis. This investigation was performed as part of her assessment (9a).
i. What is the investigation?
ii. What does it show?
iii. What are the advantages over and above CT?

9: Answer

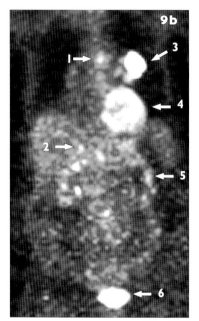

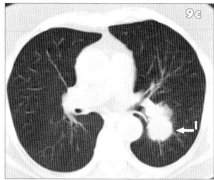

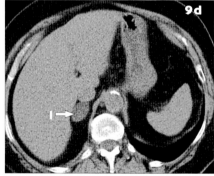

9 i. The investigation is a frontal view of a PET scan.

ii. The image demonstrates normal tracer activity in the heart, gut, and urinary bladder (**9b**, 1 abnormal mediastinal lymph node uptake; 2 abnormal right adrenal uptake; 3 left lung tumour; 4 normal cardiac uptake; 5 normal gut uptake; 6 normal urinary bladder uptake). Abnormal uptake is seen within the left lung corresponding to the tumour seen in the apical segment of the left lower lobe on CT (**9c**, 1 tumour in apical segment of left lower lobe), within a mediastinal lymph node (CT showed no abnormally enlarged lymph nodes), and also within the right adrenal gland (found to be enlarged on CT [**9d**], 1 enlarged right adrenal gland). On the basis of the imaging features, the patient was not deemed suitable for curative surgical treatment.

iii. PET uses [^{18}F]-fluorodeoxyglucose, a radiolabelled glucose analogue which is a marker for glucose metabolism and remains trapped in tumour cells after phosphorylation. The main advantage over CT is that it assesses functional activity rather than morphology. In the context of lung cancer, PET imaging has been shown to be superior to CT in demonstrating mediastinal lymph node involvement, and distant metastases. The drawbacks of PET are that other disease processes, such as infection, may show increased activity and that there may be false-negative results with pulmonary neoplasms <1 cm in diameter and slow-growing bronchioalveolar cell carcinomas.

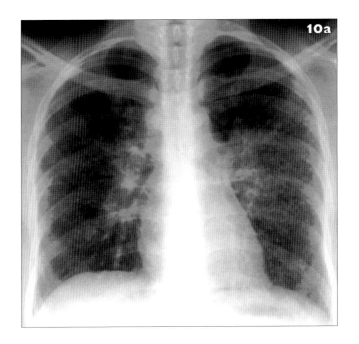

10 A 32-year-old male presented with shortness of breath, cough, and malaise while skiing at high altitude. His symptoms were attributed to high altitude pulmonary oedema. However, he made no symptomatic improvement 2 weeks following descent to sea level. He was a nonsmoker and had an unremarkable past medical history. On examination, he was well, not clubbed or cyanosed. He had widespread inspiratory crackles in both lungs. He had no skin lesions or abnormal ocular findings. Lung function tests showed a mixed restrictive and obstructive pattern. FEV_1 and FVC (predicted values): 75%; RV/TLC: 107%; DL_{CO}: 61%. Biochemical and haematological parameters were all within normal limits. His radiograph is shown (10a).

i. What is the likely radiographic diagnosis?
ii. What findings would be expected on HRCT?

10: Answer

10 i. The PA chest radiograph shows bilateral hilar and right paratracheal lymphadenopathy (**10a**). There is a widespread bilateral reticulonodular infiltrate involving all lung zones but with a mid-zone predominance. Lung volumes are normal. Appearances are typical of pulmonary sarcoidosis. The HRCT demonstrates profuse, small (1–5 mm) well-defined nodules scattered throughout all lung zones. These nodules

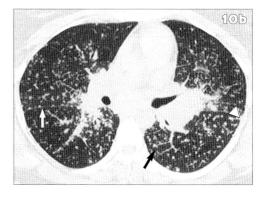

have a predilection for bronchovascular and subpleural lymphatics, reflected by bronchovascular beading (**10b**, black arrow), fissural nodularity (white arrow), and subpleural nodularity (arrowhead).

Sarcoidosis is a common multi-system disease of unknown aetiology, characterized by widespread development of noncaseating epithelioid cell granulomas. Intrathoracic manifestations are common and pulmonary involvement causes most of the morbidity and mortality. Most patients present between the ages of 20 and 40 years. Typical features at presentation include cough and dyspnoea, erythema nodosum, and ocular involvement. However, up to 50% may be asymptomatic and present with an incidental abnormal chest radiograph. Lung function tests may show a restrictive and/or obstructive pattern. Typically there is a reduced TLC, reduced gas transfer, and a restrictive ventilatory defect. The typical radiographic findings are of bilateral symmetric hilar and right paratracheal lymphadenopathy. The pattern of parenchymal involvement (which rarely occurs without lymphadenopathy) is extremely variable but the classical finding is of widespread bilateral reticulonodular shadowing, with a mid- to upper-zone predominance. The disease may progress to fibrosis which has a characteristic distribution, radiating from the hila into the mid and upper zones.

ii. Although the HRCT findings can be extremely variable (including widespread ground-glass opacification and focal areas of consolidation), the majority of cases demonstrate at least some of the typical features described above. The HRCT features include peribronchovascular interstitial thickening or nodularity (usually concentrated around the hila within the central mid and upper lungs) and small well-defined nodules which are often related to the interlobular septa and pleura. The gold standard for diagnosis has traditionally been histopathological examination of a lung biopsy (usually transbronchial) which demonstrates noncaseating epithelioid cell granulomas. However, in practice, typical clinical, functional, and radiological findings are often sufficient to make the diagnosis.

11 A 52-year-old male presented with severe abdominal pain. On examination, he was unwell and hypovolaemic. He had a past medical history of indigestion and was slightly anaemic. He was resuscitated with intravenous fluid and a right internal jugular central line was inserted.

What does the erect radiograph show (11a)?

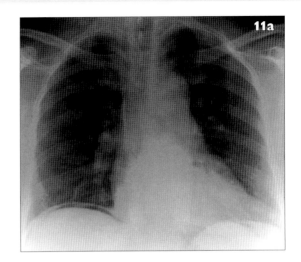

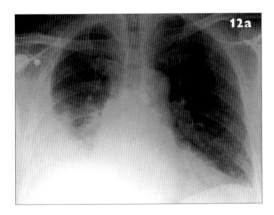

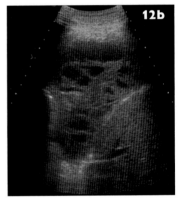

12 A 63-year-old male presented with a cough and a fever. He had been unwell for 2 weeks and despite antibiotic treatment, was not improving. He was an ex-smoker and was normally fit and well. On examination, he was not clubbed, but was pyrexial and tachycardic. The right base of the chest was dull to percussion with absent breath sounds. His blood tests showed a raised white cell count, CRP, and ESR. The chest radiograph (12a) and an ultrasound of the right chest (12b) are shown.
i. What do the examinations show?
ii. How should the diagnosis be confirmed?
iii. What is the treatment?

11, 12: Answers

11 The radiograph is a portable AP erect projection and shows the right internal jugular central venous catheter tip within the distal superior vena cava. In addition, there is a thin sliver of free intraperitoneal gas under the right hemidiaphragm (**11b**, arrows). The lungs are clear. These appearances are indicative of perforation of an intra-abdominal viscus. In this case, the cause was a peptic ulcer, but other less common causes include perforation of a diverticulum or malignant tumour.

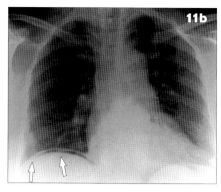

Radiographic demonstration of a pneumoperitoneum is very sensitive, with as little as 1 ml of free gas being detected on an erect chest radiograph or left lateral decubitus abdominal radiograph. The accuracy depends on careful attention to technique, however, as the patient must remain in the erect or lateral decubitus position for 5–10 minutes, to allow gas to rise to the highest position. Free gas may be more difficult to detect with certainty under the left hemidiaphragm or on a supine abdominal radiograph because of coexisting bowel gas.

12 i. The chest radiograph shows a right-sided pleural effusion with some volume loss within the right hemithorax (**12a**). The medial border of the effusion does not have the classical 'meniscus' sign (i.e. a concave upper border) and is slightly convex, raising the possibility of loculation. The ultrasound confirms a pleural effusion, containing echogenic debris and septations (**12b**). The appearances are typical for an empyema.
ii. The diagnosis of empyema can be confirmed by diagnostic aspiration.
iii. The treatment is chest tube drainage of the pleural effusion in the first instance, although sometimes patients with very heavily loculated or septated effusions (such as this case) require surgical intervention.

In the majority of patients with an empyema, there is a history of pneumonia, surgery, trauma, or subdiaphragmatic infection. The commonest organisms found in a nontuberculous empyema include *Streptococcus* species, anaerobes, and *Staphylococcus aureus*. The appearances on the chest radiograph may be of a straightforward pleural effusion with a concave upper border, but often the effusion has an unusual shape if loculations are present. On ultrasound, loculations and septations are usually evident, but in some cases none are seen. Diagnostic aspiration is necessary to distinguish empyema from a parapneumonic effusion (which resolves without intervention). CT is sometimes required in complex empyemas, to plan the optimum site of chest tube placement, and if there is no improvement after drainage. The CT features which may be seen include a lentiform or lens-shaped collection, and thickening and enhancement of both the visceral and parietal pleura post-intravenous contrast administration.

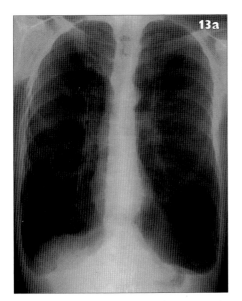
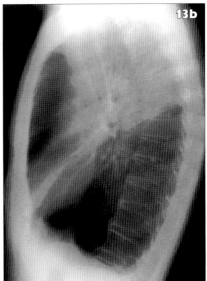

13 A 46-year-old male was referred for consideration of lung volume reduction surgery. He had become increasingly short of breath over the previous 10 years and had had approximately eight infective exacerbations per year, requiring treatment with corticosteroids as well as antibiotics. He had a family history of respiratory problems and had worked as an electrician. He was an ex-smoker (10 pack-years) and had stopped 4 years earlier. He was not breathless at rest but had a barrel-shaped chest with very quiet breath sounds throughout. Lung function tests (predicted values) showed a severe obstructive defect with air trapping: FEV_1: 15%; FVC: 44.5%; TLC: 142%; RV: 353%; TL_{CO}: 20%; K_{CO}: 29% of predicted, respectively. The full blood count, urea and electrolytes and liver function tests were normal.

i. What do the PA and lateral chest radiographs (13a, b) show ?

ii. Could all these abnormalities be attributable to smoking?

13: Answer

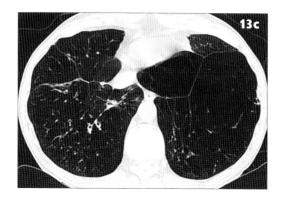

13 i. The chest radiographs show large volume lungs with an increased AP diameter of the chest on the lateral view (13a, b). There is paucity of pulmonary vasculature especially in the lower zones and bronchial wall thickening. A CT scan of the thorax confirmed widespread panacinar (or panlobular) emphysema with lower zone predominance (13c). Dilated, thickened airways, with some mucus plugging were seen in the lower lobes, indicating mild cylindrical bronchiectasis. These finding were supportive of a diagnosis of emphysema secondary to alpha-1-antitrypsin (AAT) deficiency. AAT level was <0.3 g/l (normal 1.8–3g/l). Subsequently, his phenotype was found to be homozygous PiZ.

ii. AAT deficiency is a rare congenital disorder, which is inherited as an autosomal dominant gene. AAT is a protease inhibitor synthesized in the liver and inhibits proteases and elastases, which are released by macrophages during inflammatory reactions, thus preventing tissue damage. Diagnosis is made by serum measurement of the enzyme and by the characteristic electophoretic mobility of the glycoprotein: medium (M) is normal, slow (S) and very slow (Z) are abnormal. Homozygotes with phenotype PiZZ are most severely affected. The incidence is 1:5000 births and most affected individuals develop lung disease with an onset of symptoms between 35 and 50 years of age (earlier in smokers). The deficiency leads to panacinar emphysema with generalized alveolar wall destruction. This effect is potentiated by cigarette smoking. Liver disease can also be a feature, presenting as cholestatic jaundice in neonates or chronic liver disease in adults.

Up to 50% of AAT deficient patients have been reported to present with chronic bronchitis. HRCT studies have confirmed airway abnormalities with bronchial wall thickening and widespread bronchiectasis (occurring in 40% of patients).

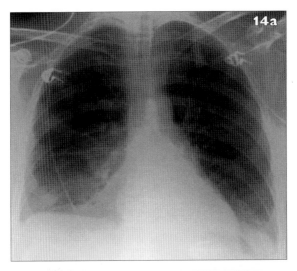

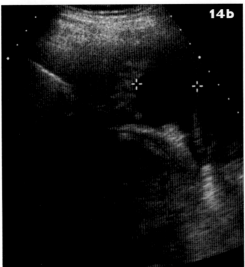

14 The radiograph of a 72- year-old male who was ventilated on the intensive care unit after having had an emergency abdominal aortic aneursym repair is shown (14a). It was proving difficult to wean him from the ventilator. Another investigation was performed in view of the radiographic appearances at the right base (14b).
i. What does the chest radiograph show?
ii. What second investigation was performed and what does it show?

14: Answer

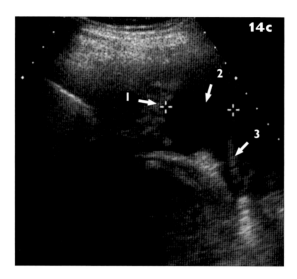

14 i. The chest radiograph shows an endotracheal tube and an apparently elevated right hemidiaphragm (14a). There is also obscuration of the medial portion of the left hemidiaphragm due to left lower lobe atelectasis. The 'peak' or highest point of the right hemidiaphragm is also seen more laterally than normal. The medial slope of the diaphragm is gradual, whereas the lateral one is steep. What appears to be the right costophrenic angle is blunted. The radiographic features are those of a subpulmonic pleural effusion.

ii. The diagnosis may be confirmed by a decubitus radiograph or, as in this instance, ultrasonography (14b, c: 1 collapsed lung; 2 pleural fluid; 3 diaphragm). The pleural fluid was subsequently drained and the patient successfully weaned from the ventilator. Pleural effusions following abdominal surgery are relatively common and occur more frequently after upper abdominal rather than lower abdominal surgery. Post-operative pulmonary atelectasis may also be a contributing factor. For reasons that are not entirely clear, pleural fluid may collect in a predominantly subpulmonic distribution, rather than throughout the pleural cavity. Subpulmonic effusions are more commonly right-sided. These types of pleural effusion may be easy to overlook as the upper edge of the fluid mimics the hemidiaphragmatic contour. However, the clue to the diagnosis is the more lateral than normal 'peak' of the hemidiaphragm.

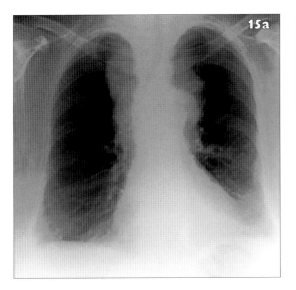
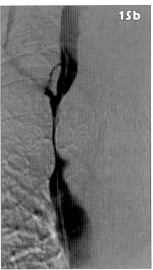

15 A 62-year-old female presented with facial and upper limb swelling, head-aches, and difficulty breathing. She had been a heavy smoker for 40 years. On examination, she was clubbed, and had facial and bilateral upper limb oedema. She was cyanosed and her eyes were suffused. She had visibly dilated upper limb and anterior chest wall veins. Her chest radiograph is shown (15a), and an image from an interventional procedure (15b).

i. What is the likely clinical diagnosis, and what are the possible causes?

ii. What does the chest radiograph show?

iii. What was the interventional procedure?

15: Answer

15 i. The likely clinical diagnosis is superior vena cava obstruction. The possible causes include carcinoma of the bronchus, metastatic carcinoma (e.g. breast), lymphoma, aortic aneurysm, or mediastinal fibrosis.

ii. The chest radiograph shows widening of the superior mediastinum due to a mediastinal mass (15a).

iii. A venogram shows marked narrowing of the superior vena cava due to extrinsic compression (15b). The interventional procedure was insertion of a radiologically-guided stent via the right femoral vein (15c). A subsequent CT shows extensive abnormal soft tissue in the superior mediastinum surrounding the great vessels (15d, 1 anterior chest wall venous collaterals; 2 enlarged internal mammary veins; 3 enlarged superior intercostal vein; 4 stent in superior vena cava; 5 abnormal mediastinal soft tissue). The CT shows the typical features of extensive venous collaterals of the anterior chest wall and hypertrophied internal mammary and superior intercostal veins. The mediastinal mass was subsequently biopsied under ultrasound guidance and a histopathological diagnosis of small cell lung cancer was made.

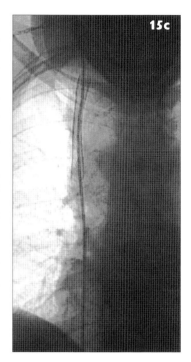

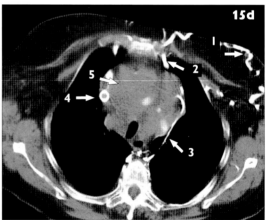

16 A 66-year-old male presented with slight breathlessness on exertion. His symptoms had started at the age of 64 years, necessitating retirement from coal mining. He also complained of a nonproductive cough. He was a heavy smoker. He kept no pets and there was no other relevant past medical history.

What does his chest radiograph (16) show?

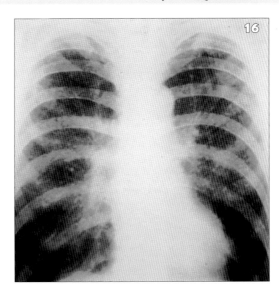

17 A 37-year-old male hairdresser presented with a cough and an abnormal chest radiograph (not shown). He had been a smoker for many years (including smoking cannabis). Otherwise he was fit and well and did not have any risk factors for HIV. His lung function tests were normal. An HRCT was performed (17a, b).
i. What does it show?
ii. What is the diagnosis?

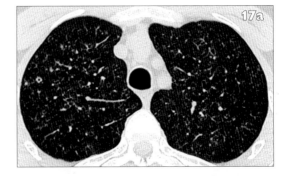

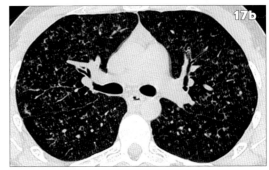

16, 17: Answers

16 The chest radiograph shows bilateral, small (2–3 mm) diameter, well-defined pulmonary nodules (**16**). A mid- and upper-zone predominance is noted. In an individual with previous heavy exposure to coal dust, the findings are those of simple coal worker's pneumoconiosis. Simple coal worker's pneumoconiosis and silicosis are often considered together as the radiological features are similar. There is often cross-contamination of dusts in mining and many coal workers are also exposed to significant quantities of silica as well as coal dust. Simple coal worker's pneumoconiosis is not usually associated with symptoms or a functional deficit. However, most workers have also been heavy smokers and may have emphysema and chronic bronchitis in addition. There is also evidence that emphysema is associated with both coal and silica dust exposure, independent of the smoking history.

The HRCT appearances of coal worker's pneumoconiosis are centrilobular nodules (adjacent to the structures in the centre of the secondary pulmonary lobule) or subpleural nodules of varying size. A small percentage of nodules calcify, increasing their conspicuity on the radiograph and HRCT.

17 i. The HRCT shows the typical features of pulmonary Langerhan's cell histiocytosis (PLCH) (**17a, b**). There is a combination of small nodules and multiple small, irregularly-shaped cystic spaces with a mid- and upper-zone predominance. Typically, there is relative sparing of the costophrenic recesses and the anterior tips of the right middle lobe and lingula. Serial HRCT studies show a progression of nodules to cavities and then cysts, with end-stage disease showing extensive parenchymal destruction which can closely resemble emphysema.

ii. The main HRCT differential is lymphangioleiomyomatosis (LAM). However, in LAM the cysts tend to be more regular in shape, uniformly scattered throughout the lungs and involving the costophrenic recesses. Nodules are not a feature of LAM. Also LAM occurs almost exclusively in females of child-bearing age.

The characteristic radiographic features of PLCH (**17c**) are a widespread nodular or reticulonodular infiltrate, often with mid- or upper-zone predominance and sparing of the costophrenic angles. The lung volumes are preserved or increased. Over 90% of affected individuals are smokers, and there seems to be no gender difference, although it was initially thought to be a commoner disease in males. Pneumothorax is a frequent complication and may be a presenting feature (**17c**, arrow).

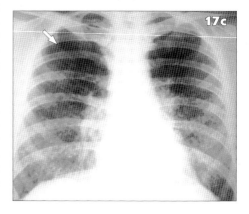

18 A 34-year-old female presented with exercise-related wheeze which required oral steroids. She subsequently had an episode of myalgia and systemic upset, again requiring oral steroids. This pattern of intermittent episodes of fever, myalgia, malaise, and wheeze had continued over 1 year. She kept no pets although there was a family history of asthma and COPD. She was not breathless at rest. She had no clubbing or lymphadenopathy. A low-grade pyrexia was noted when she was unwell. Eosinophils were 20% of peripheral white cell count and the ESR was 57 mm/hr. Skin tests and fungal precipitins were negative. Autoantibodies were also negative. Serum immunoglobulins were normal. Sputum was sterile but large numbers of eosinophils were present. Two radiographs are shown (18a, b) which were taken 6 months apart.
i. What do they show?
ii. What is the likely diagnosis?

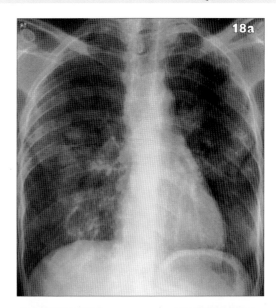

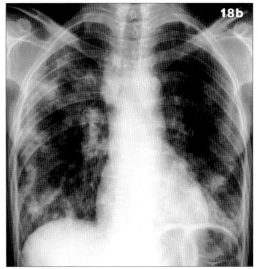

18: Answer

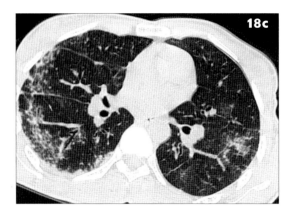

18 i. The initial chest radiograph shows patchy bilateral areas of consolidation both peripherally and centrally located but with a mid-zone predominance (18a). The subsequent radiograph shows a predominantly peripheral distribution of consolidation, with new areas at the left base, and other areas that have resolved (e.g. centrally within the right mid zone) (18b). There is also right paratracheal lymphadenopathy on the later radiograph.

ii. The clinical and radiographic features in this patient are compatible with the diagnosis of chronic eosinophilic pneumonia. Chronic eosinophilic pneumonia often develops in middle age. The male to female ratio is 1:2. Fifty percent of individuals are atopic and 40% are asthmatic. Symptoms of malaise, marked weight loss, spiking fever, drenching night sweats, and dyspnoea with productive cough may be misdiagnosed as TB. This may be reinforced by the chest radiographic appearances. The ESR and eosinophil count are elevated in the majority. The serum IgE is borderline or normal, in contrast to allergic bronchopulmonary aspergillosis (ABPA) or parasitic pulmonary eosinophilia, in which it is significantly raised. Pathologically, there is an eosinophil-rich exudate in the alveoli and interstitium. Histological features of organizing pneumonia or low-grade vasculitis may also be present. Radiographically, peripheral, nonsegmental, homogeneous consolidation with or without air bronchograms is seen in two-thirds of patients. The upper zones are affected more than the middle zones, followed by the lower zones. The consolidation comes and goes spontaneously and sometimes recurs in the same location. The characteristic peripheral distribution is evident on the radiograph in approximately 50% of cases. The distribution on the radiograph may be random, central, or a combination of central and peripheral. Pleural effusions and cavitation are rare. CT typically shows predominantly peripheral multifocal consolidation and/or ground-glass opacity (18c). CT demonstrates a peripheral predominance even when this is not apparent on the radiograph and helps to confirm the diagnosis.

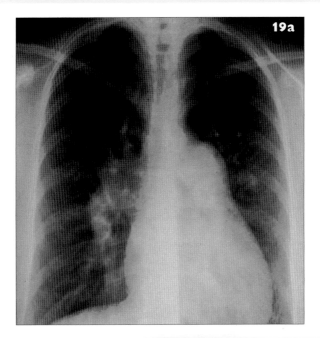

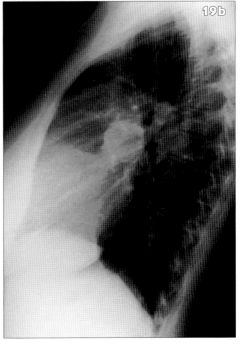

19 A 31-year-old female had a history of gradual progressive shortness of breath and decreased exercise tolerance. She had no relevant past medical history and was not taking any medication. She was not clubbed or cyanosed. Her lungs were clear on auscultation but a loud pulmonary second sound was noted at cardiac examination. An ECG showed right bundle branch block and right ventricular strain. A chest radiograph (PA and left lateral, 19a, b) was performed.

i. What are the radiographic findings?

ii. What further investigations should be performed?

19: Answer

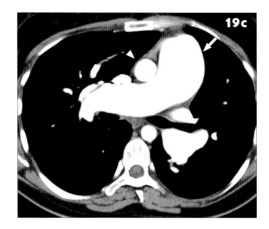

19 i. The PA chest radiograph shows cardiomegaly and an enlarged pulmonary outflow tract and central pulmonary arteries (**19a**). The lateral radiograph confirms the enlargement of the central pulmonary arteries (**19b**). There is tapering of arteries and the peripheral lung appears oligaemic. The appearances are those of pulmonary arterial hypertension.

ii. Transthoracic echocardiography is used as a screening test to estimate the tricuspid valve regurgitant flow velocity, as an indirect measure of pulmonary arterial pressure. However, direct pressure measurements at cardiac catheterization are more accurate. Pressure measurements at cardiac catheterization confirmed the diagnosis in the current case with a high pulmonary vascular resistance, no evidence of a left-to-right shunt, and normal pulmonary wedge pressure. Further investigation should include ventilation-perfusion scintigraphy or a CT pulmonary angiogram (CTPA) to exclude chronic thromboembolic disease. An image from the CTPA shows the enlarged central pulmonary artery (**19c**, arrow) which should normally be approximately the same diameter as the ascending thoracic aorta (arrowhead). In this case, there was no evidence of chronic thromboembolic disease and no other clinically discernible cause of pulmonary hypertension, such as underlying lung disease or left-to-right shunt. A diagnosis of primary pulmonary hypertension was made.

The aetiology of primary pulmonary hypertension is uncertain, although various theories have been suggested. Pathologically, there is fibromuscular intimal hypertrophy which results in narrowing and obliteration of the lumen of blood vessels, usually the precapillary arteries. Medical treatments include intravenous prostacyclin and inhaled nitric oxide, although some patients ultimately require heart–lung transplantation.

20 A 46-year-old male presented with long-standing productive cough throughout childhood and limited exercise tolerance. He had had a recent episode of right heart failure requiring admission. Symptoms had been worse in the last few years, with more copious sputum production and episodes of pleuritic chest pain with chest wall tenderness. Past medical history included previous sinus surgery. His sister had also had similar symptoms. On examination, he was clubbed with bilateral fine inspiratory crepitations. There was no evidence of cardiac failure. Blood tests showed polycythaemia and arterial hypoxia. Serum immunoglobulins and alpha-1-antitrypsin levels were normal.

i. What do the chest radiograph and sinus view (20a, b) show?

ii. What is the unifying diagnosis?

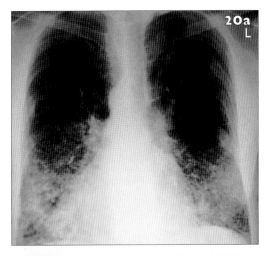

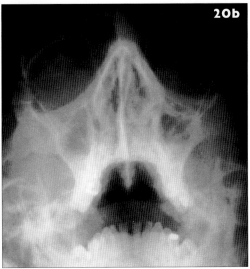

20: Answer

20 i. The chest radiograph demonstrates dextrocardia with a right-sided aortic arch (20a). There are ring opacities of varying sizes bilaterally, some of which contain fluid levels, predominantly in the mid and lower zones. There is upper lobe blood flow distribution, reflecting shunting of blood due to the severe lower lobe disease. Multiple fractured ribs at various stages of healing are demonstrated due to repetitive coughing. There are fluid levels within both maxillary antra consistent with sinusitis (20b).

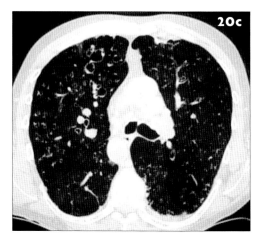

ii. The unifying diagnosis is Kartagener's syndrome. This syndrome consists of situs inversus, paranasal sinusitis, and bronchiectasis. It is a subset of ciliary dyskinesia syndrome, in which a variety of genetically determined defects in ciliary function interfere with mucociliary clearance, leading to recurrent upper and lower respiratory tract infections. In this case the cilia beat frequency was 9 Hz (normal range 10–20 Hz). There is autosomal recessive inheritance and an equal sex incidence.

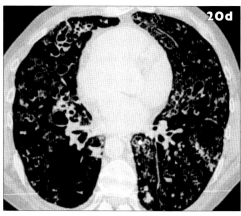

Males are usually infertile whereas female fertility is usually unaffected. Bronchiectasis develops in childhood and adolescence. Prognosis is good and life expectancy is generally not shortened. The HRCT demonstrates widespread cystic bronchiectasis (20c, d). The left lung has anatomic right-sided configuration and *vice versa*.

21 An 80-year-old female presented with a 2-week history of productive cough, not responding to antibiotics. On examination, she was apyrexial, not clubbed, and with a normal respiratory rate. She had seen her family doctor for similar symptoms several times in the preceding year. She had been a smoker in the past but had given up 20 years ago. She lived alone and kept a budgerigar. Her urea and electrolytes were normal, her white cell count was slightly raised, as were the ESR and CRP.

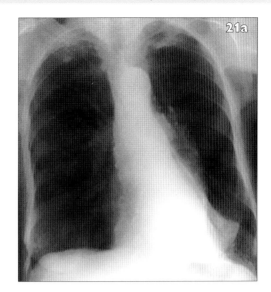

i. What does the chest radiograph show (21a)?
ii. What imaging investigation should be performed next?

22 A 69-year-old male presented with a history of haemoptysis. On examination, he was apyrexial but clubbed and cachexic. His full blood count and urea and electrolytes were normal.

i. What does the chest radiograph (22) show?
ii. What is the likely diagnosis?
iii. Can the cause be identified on the radiograph?

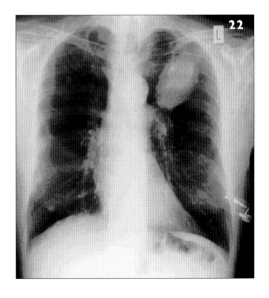

21, 22: Answers

21 i. The chest radiograph shows a triangular-shaped density behind the left side of the heart, with obscuration of the medial contour of the left hemidiaphragm (21a). There is also volume loss within the left hemithorax and the mediastinum appears deviated to the left. There is unfolding of the thoracic aorta. There is an incidental calcific density at the right apex. The appearances are those of a left lower lobe collapse.

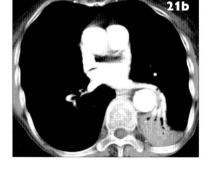

ii. In a patient with a clinical picture of a nonresolving lower respiratory tract infection, an endobronchial lesion needs to be excluded and the next imaging investigation of choice is a CT. A bronchoscopy was also performed.

The CT shows the collapsed left lower lobe (21b). The atelectatic lung demonstrates enhancement on these intravenous contrast-enhanced images. The collapsed lower lobe is draped across the descending aorta, giving rise to a convex outer border to the collapse. This appearance can give the erroneous impression of an underlying mass on radiography, although the CT readily demonstrates the cause of the convex border to be due to the descending thoracic aorta, not an underlying mass. Air bronchograms are seen within the collapsed lower lobe, which is against the presence of a central obstructing lesion within the lower lobe bronchus. However, this sign does not always completely exclude a central lesion. No endobronchial lesion was demonstrated on CT (confirmed on bronchoscopy).

22 i. The chest radiograph shows an approximately 4 cm diameter mass within the left upper zone (22). The margins are well defined. There is a small fleck of calcification projected over the density. The left hilum appears bulky, suggestive of hilar lymphadenopathy. Several small nodules (<1 cm in diameter) are present in the right lung. The lungs are of large volume, indicating obstructive lung disease.

ii. The likely diagnosis is a bronchogenic carcinoma with left hilar lymphadenopathy and contralateral pulmonary metastases.

iii. The cause is likely to be due to cigarette smoking (note the patient's cigarette lighter in his left shirt pocket!), also resulting in emphysema.

Lung cancer is the most common fatal cancer in men and women. The major cause of disease is cigarette smoking, with other factors (e.g. asbestos exposure) also implicated. The disease tends to be relatively asymptomatic until late, when patients present with cough, wheezing, haemoptysis, recurrent pneumonia, or paraneoplastic syndromes. The majority of patients present with advanced disease, too late for curative surgery. Contraindications to surgery include distant metastases, e.g. to the contralateral lung (as in this case). The common histological types are squamous cell carcinoma, adenocarcinoma, large cell anaplastic carcinoma, and small (oat) cell carcinoma.

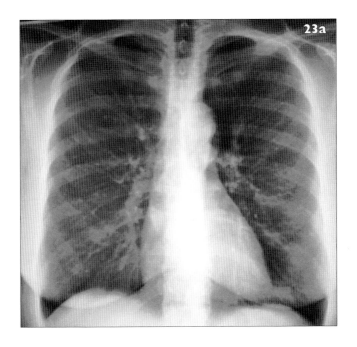

23 A 23-year-old female presented for a pre-immigration chest radiograph. She was normally fit and well and had no symptoms.
i. What does the chest radiograph show (23a)?
ii. What investigation should be performed next?

23: Answer

23 i. The PA chest radiograph shows a smooth, well-defined curvilinear opacity in the aortopulmonary region (**23b**, arrows). It does not obscure the left hilum or the descending thoracic aorta. The CT shows the lesion to lie within the posterior mediastinum, adjacent to the descending thoracic aorta (**23c**, arrows). It is of soft tissue attenuation on these unenhanced images, with no areas of calcification. Intravenous contrast was not given due to a previous contrast reaction. There is no adjacent rib abnormality and no apparent widening of the adjacent neural foramen is seen.

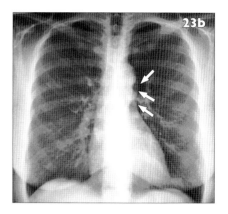

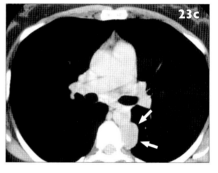

The differential diagnosis of a posterior mediastinal mass in adults in a paravertebral location includes neural tumours (e.g. neurofibroma), extramedullary haematopoiesis, an abscess (often with disc space and vertebral body destruction) and metastases (bone destruction with preserved disc spaces). In the current case, there is no evidence of bone destruction.

ii. The next investigation of choice is an MRI (not shown), which demonstrated the typical dumb-bell extension of the mass into the adjacent neural foramina, typical of a neurofibroma. She was followed up for 2 years with no radiographic change.

Neural tumours are often well-defined, spherical lesions with a smooth or lobulated outline. It is not possible to differentiate benign from malignant tumours when they are localized. They are normally situated in the posterior mediastinum in the paravertebral region, unless there is involvement of the vagus or phrenic nerves. Calcification may be a feature, but is relatively rare in nerve sheath tumours. The pressure effects on adjacent bony structures are a useful sign in benign neural tumours, with splaying or scalloping of the ribs without bony cortex destruction. Large tumours may be associated with scoliosis. The intervertebral foramina may also be widened. Neural tumours may show heterogeneous attenuation on CT, with low attenuation areas due to cystic degeneration. The lesions are often vascular and may demonstrate avid contrast enhancement on CT. MRI is superior to CT at demonstrating intraspinal extension.

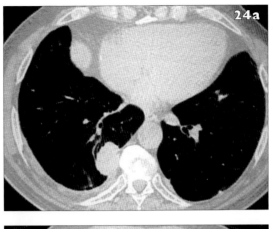

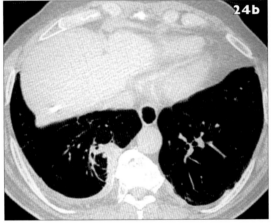

24 A 73-year-old male presented after a new shadow was seen on his chest radiograph (not shown) 2 years after coronary artery bypass grafting. The postoperative period had been complicated by bilateral pleural effusions requiring intercostal chest tube drainage and prolonged chest pain which had resolved with analgesia. He had been exposed to asbestos in the past. On examination, he was well. His lung function tests showed a mild reduction in lung volumes with a normal DL_{CO} and a transfer coefficient (K_{CO}) 115% of the predicted value. Two HRCT images are shown, **24a** being the image immediately superior to **24b**.
i. What do the HRCT images show?
ii. What is the diagnosis?

24: Answer

24 i. The HRCT shows a 3.5 cm × 3 cm soft tissue attenuation lesion in the right lower lobe posteriorly. The broncho-vascular structures appear 'swirled' and the mass has an appearance similar to a 'comet's tail' inferiorly (24c, arrowhead). The lesion contacts an area of diffuse pleural thickening and there is volume loss in the right lower lobe, as denoted by the posterior displacement of the oblique fissure (arrow). There are some pleural plaques on the left in the para-vertebral region.

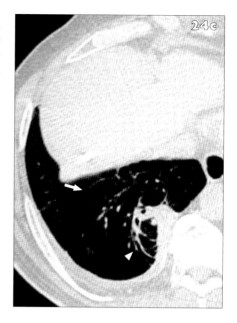

ii. The CT features are those of folded lung or rounded atelectasis. Folded lung refers to peripheral atelectatic lung adjacent to an area of pleural thickening, with characteristic drawing in of the bronchi and vessels into the atelectatic lung. Synonyms for folded lung include Blesovsky's syndrome, rounded atelec-tasis, atelectatic pseudotumour, and pulmonary pseudotumour. Blesovsky first reported three cases in 1966 in which there was unusually extensive lung folding due to a fibrous membrane on the costal surface of the visceral pleura of the lower lobe, and he termed it 'folded lung'. There is a strong association with previous asbestos exposure but any cause of an organizing pleural exudate such as tuberculosis, histoplasmosis, Dressler's syndrome, following cardiac surgery, and haemothorax may be responsible.

On chest radiography, folded lung appears as a rounded peripheral pulmonary mass; distortion of the adjacent lung may or may not be obvious and pleural thickening is usually evident. The lesion may be mistaken for a bronchogenic carcinoma on radiography but CT is most helpful in making the diagnosis and usually obviates the need for biopsy. The major CT features are: (1) rounded or oval mass (2.5–7 cm in diameter) abutting a peripheral pleural surface; (2) the curving 'comet tail' of bronchovascular structures converging towards the mass; (3) thickening of the adjacent pleura; and (4) evidence of volume loss in the adjacent lung, as demonstrated by the posterior displacement of the oblique fissure in the current case.

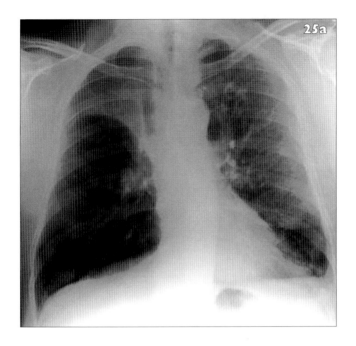

25 A 71-year-old male presented with a 1-month history of progressive shortness of breath on exertion and a cough, productive of white sputum. His past medical history included probable tuberculosis (TB) during the Second World War. He was a smoker, averaging 6 cigarettes per day for many years. On examination, he was dyspnoeic on minimal exertion but there was no cyanosis or clubbing. There was decreased air entry over the right apex. The chest was otherwise clear to auscultation.

i. What does the chest radiograph show (25a)?
ii. What further investigations should be performed?

25: Answer

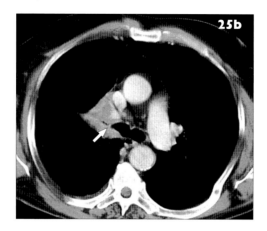

25 i. The chest radiograph shows increased density in the right upper zone with elevation and concavity of the horizontal fissure (25a). The radiographic features are those of a collapsed right upper lobe. There are some healed fractured ribs on the left. There are calcified mediastinal lymph nodes and some scarring within the left upper zone, consistent with the patient's previous history of TB. No other focal pulmonary lesions are identified. The most common causes of lobar collapse in adults are bronchial neoplasm and mucus plugs. As volume loss occurs, the right upper lobe collapses superiorly, anteriorly, and medially. The middle lobe expands superiorly and laterally, occupying the area lateral to the collapsed upper lobe. The right lower lobe expands superiorly and posteriorly, occupying the area posterior to the collapsed upper lobe. When a lobe collapses due to a large central obstructing mass, the central portion of the collapsed lobe may drape over the mass causing a convex bulge. This appearance is known as the S sign of Golden, and is highly suggestive of a proximal bronchogenic carcinoma. This sign can be appreciated on a frontal radiograph in collapse of the right upper lobe, right lower lobe, and left lower lobe, and on a lateral radiograph in collapse of the right middle lobe and left upper lobe.
ii. The next investigations of choice are CT and bronchoscopy. The CT shows a soft tissue mass at the right hilum around the right main bronchus which is narrowing the orifice to the right upper lobe (25b, arrow). The signs of lobar collapse can be equally seen on CT. The collapsed right upper lobe typically appears as a triangular soft tissue density lying against the mediastinum and anterior chest wall on CT. Upward displacement of the right upper lobe bronchus causes reorientation of the bronchial anatomy, with the bronchus intermedius moving laterally and the right middle lobe bronchus displaced anteriorly and reorientated into a more horizontal position. Biopsy of the lesion showed a squamous cell carcinoma on histopathological examination of the sample.

26 A 61-year-old male complained of shortness of breath and a long history of chronic low back pain which limited his mobility. He had been fairly well until 4 years ago, when he developed progressive shortness of breath. He was a nonsmoker with no significant occupational history. There was no history of keeping household pets. He was diagnosed as having asthma but did not respond to inhaled or oral steroids.

On examination, the patient was slightly tachypnoeic. There was no cyanosis or clubbing. Auscultation of the lungs did not reveal any significant findings. Lung function tests showed diminished diffusion capacity. ECG demonstrated 'p' pulmonale with right axis deviation. Serum protein C and protein S were not deficient. Doppler ultrasound of the veins in the lower limbs showed no evidence of deep venous thrombosis. Spiral CT pulmonary angiography was performed (26a–c).

i. What are the findings?
ii. What is the likely cause of the patient's symptoms?

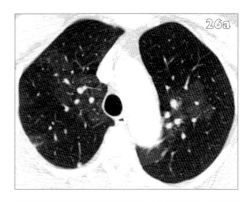

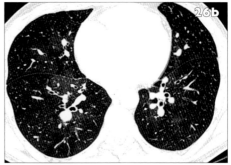

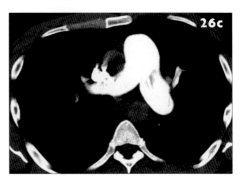

26: Answer

26 i. CT sections on lung windows show a mosaic perfusion pattern, with inhomogeneity of the lung density (**26a, b**). The pulmonary vasculature in the areas of decreased lung attenuation appears of decreased calibre compared with the vessels in the relatively dense lungs. The main pulmonary trunk and proximal pulmonary arteries at the hila are enlarged, reflecting underlying pulmonary hypertension. There are filling defects within the main pulmonary arteries which have a 'web-like' configuration (**26c**) as opposed to the more defined filling defects seen in acute pulmonary embolism (see Question **69**). A linear filling defect is also seen within a segmental artery within the left upper lobe (**26c**). The appearances are consistent with chronic pulmonary thromboembolism.

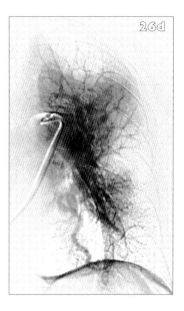

ii. The HRCT appearance of inhomogeneity in attenuation of the lung parenchyma is nonspecific. The so called 'mosaic attenuation pattern' can be seen in small airway disease, pulmonary vascular disease, and infiltrative lung disease. In chronic pulmonary thromboembolic disease, the CT mosaic pattern is due to regions of hyperaemic lung (higher attenuation) seen adjacent to areas of oligaemic lung (lower attenuation). When mosaic attenuation is due to small airway disease and pulmonary vascular disease, the pulmonary vessels in the low attenuation areas are smaller compared with those in the more opaque lung. The reduction in vessel calibre is due to reflex vasoconstriction in small airway disease, and a combination of vasoconstriction and occlusion in thromboembolic disease. When the cause of the mosaic pattern is an infiltrative process, the vessels are usually similar in size in areas of differing attenuation. End-expiratory scans may be helpful in distinguishing between these groups of diseases. Differences in lung attenuation resulting from small airway disease are greatly accentuated on end-expiratory HRCT scans.

In patients with chronic thromboembolic disease, the commonest CT and radiographic finding is a dilated pulmonary trunk. The diameter of the pulmonary trunk shows good correlation with the mean pulmonary arterial pressure. Other CT features include dilatation of the right ventricle and deviation of the interventricular septum. Intra-arterial filling defects such as webs and concentric or laminated clot are also seen. A conventional selective left pulmonary angiogram on the same patient shows occlusion of segmental pulmonary arteries resulting in abnormalities of regional perfusion, leading to relatively hypovascular areas (**26d**).

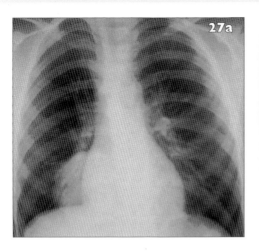

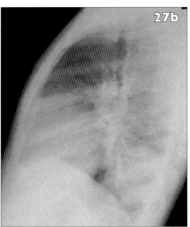

27 An 8-year-old child presented with fever and cough productive of green sputum. He was normally fit and well, with no similar episodes previously. On examination, he was pyrexial but his chest was clear on auscultation. His white cell count was raised (neutrophilia), but otherwise blood tests were normal. PA and lateral chest radiographs were performed (27a, b).
i. What are the findings?
ii. What is the likely diagnosis?
iii. What further investigations (if any) should be suggested?

28 The chest radiograph is shown of a 72-year-old male (28a).

What is the most likely diagnosis?

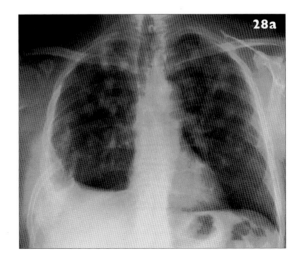

27, 28: Answers

27 i. The PA and lateral chest radiographs demonstrate a rounded opacity which lies posteriorly within the right lower lobe (27a, b). It appears to contact the pleural surface posteriorly (27c). On the lateral radiograph, there is the impression of an air bronchogram (27c, arrows).

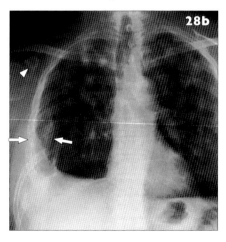

ii. These findings, together with the clinical history, are suggestive of a rounded pneumonia. A repeat radiograph was obtained 1 month later and showed complete resolution after antibiotic treatment.

Rounded pneumonias often appear very 'mass-like' on radiographs, but the clinical history is the clue to the diagnosis in this case. This pattern of pneumonia is seen more commonly in children than in adults and is usually due to pneumococcus.

iii. No other investigations, apart from a repeat radiograph in some cases, are required if the child responds well to treatment and it is the first presentation.

28 The chest radiograph shows multiple, well-defined, bilateral pulmonary nodules thoughout both lungs. They are 1–2 cm in diameter. The lateral aspect of the right sixth rib is abnormal, with loss of the cortex and increased soft tissue related to this region (28b, arrows). There is a right-sided pleural reaction with blunting of the costophrenic angle. Note also that most of the right scapula is missing, leaving only the coracoid process (28b, arrowhead). The most likely diagnosis is of widespread malignancy with multiple pulmonary and bony metastases. The primary malignancy in this case was a renal cell carcinoma. It is unusual to see sparing of lower zones as in this case.

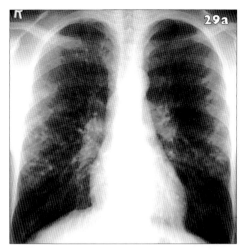

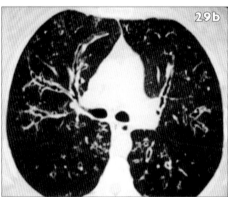

29 A 23-year-old male with a known chronic lung disease was referred for assessment for heart–lung transplantation. He was diagnosed at the age of 18 months. He remained relatively stable throughout his childhood and early teens but in the last few years had developed increasingly severe respiratory symptoms and weight loss, requiring multiple hospital admissions. He required continuous oxygen (2 l/min via nasal prongs) and his exercise tolerance had fallen so that he could now manage only 2–3 stairs without stopping. On examination, he was clubbed but not cyanosed (on 2 l/min O_2). There were widespread crackles throughout both lungs. Lung function tests showed a markedly reduced FEV_1 and FVC. The TLC was preserved with a reduced DL_{CO}. He was hypoxic on air with a raised pCO_2.

What findings are present on the chest radiograph and HRCT (**29a, b**)?

29: Answer

29 The radiograph shows the typical features of cystic fibrosis (CF) including hyperinflation, bronchiectasis (ring shadows, tramlines, and fluid levels within bronchiectatic airways), bronchial wall thickening, and hilar enlargement (**29a**). These features are most prominent in the upper and mid zones. Hilar enlargement may be due to pulmonary arterial hypertension and lymphadenopathy. The HRCT shows the full spectrum of severe bronchiectatic changes with cystic, varicose, and cylindrical bronchiectasis (**29b**). Although all lung zones are involved, the upper lobes are typically most severely affected. There is widespread mosaic attenuation indicating coexisting small airways obliteration.

CF is the most common inherited lethal disorder in the Caucasian population, with an incidence ranging from 1:2500 (USA) to 1:500 (Scotland). The autosomal recessive disorder is caused by a single deletion in a gene (DF508) on chromosome 7 in approximately 70–75% of cases. The remaining cases are accounted for by more than 400 different mutations. Expression of the CF gene is restricted to epithelial cells and results in abnormal chloride ion transport. This causes an increased salt concentration in the sweat and is the principle behind the diagnostic sweat test. The majority of cases present in infancy with recurrent chest infections and failure to thrive. Over two-thirds of cases are diagnosed by the age of 1 year. Nevertheless, patients may present in adulthood.

Pulmonary complications account for the majority of the morbidity and mortality. The mucus of patients with CF is more viscous than normal. This results in decreased mucociliary clearance and encourages bacterial colonization. The initial colonizing organisms are *Staphylococcus aureus* and *Haemophilus influenzae*. These cause inflammation and injury to the small airways, creating an environment favourable for colonization by *Pseudomonas aeruginosa*, which causes chronic infection in up to 90% of patients.

Complications include pneumothorax, believed to be due to rupture of subpleural blebs, and colonization with *Aspergillus fumigatus*, which may result in mycetoma formation in a pre-existing bronchiectatic cystic cavity. The incidence of allergic bronchopulmonary aspergillosis increases with age and is a relatively common cause of extensive consolidation in patients with CF. Super-added infection may occur with *Mycobacterium* sp. and viruses. Haemoptysis is common due to chronic inflammation causing friable mucosa and bronchial artery hypertrophy. The development of cor pulmonale is associated with a poor prognosis.

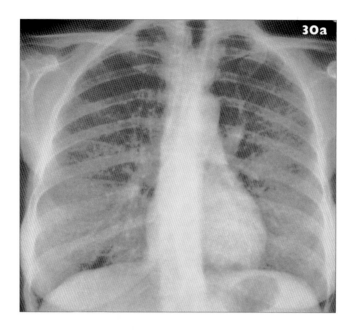

30 A 37-year-old female presented with a 1-month history of night time cough and wheeze. She had been treated by her family doctor for an acute respiratory tract infection 1 month prior to presentation and had made a good recovery. She kept fantail pigeons. On examination, she had widespread inspiratory and expiratory crackles and wheeze. Lung function tests showed a restrictive ventilatory defect with an FEV$_1$ of 77% predicted, an FVC of 77% predicted, and a marked reduction in the gas transfer factor (DL$_{CO}$) (42% predicted). Serology for mycoplasma, *Legionella* sp., cytomegalovirus, and *Aspergillus* sp. were all negative. Avian precipitins were strongly positive to pigeon and budgerigar sera.

i. What does the chest radiograph show (30a)?

ii. What is the likely diagnosis?

iii. What might HRCT show?

30: Answer

30 i. The admission chest radiograph demonstrates normal lung volumes and a subtle widespread ground-glass opacity (30a).

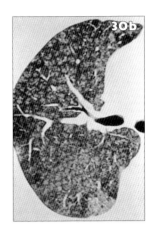

ii. The likely diagnosis is subacute extrinsic allergic alveolitis (also known as hypersensitivity pneumonitis).
iii. The typical HRCT features consist of widespread ground-glass opacification with ill-defined centrilobular nodules (30b). The other features are a so-called mosaic attenuation pattern (due to geographic areas of increased and decreased attenuation) (30c), which is accentuated on end-expiratory images (30d) due to air-trapping.

Extrinsic allergic alveolitis is a complex immuno-logical reaction by the lungs to inhaled organic antigens.

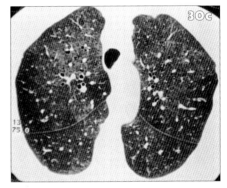

A large number of causal antigens have been identified, but the commonest are fungal spores in mouldy hay resulting in farmer's lung, or bird droppings and feathers giving rise to bird fancier's disease. Extrinsic allergic alveolitis is divided into acute, subacute, and chronic disease depending on the length of exposure and quantity of inhaled antigen. Each stage has distinctive pathological features, although co-existence of more than one stage in an individual patient is common. It is rare to image patients in the acute phase, as symptoms are often short-lived and wane spontaneously on cessation of exposure to the antigen. More often, patients present with subacute disease, and the common radiographic features are diffuse ground-glass opacification or a subtle reticulonodular pattern, but the radiograph may also be normal. The history, clinical findings and serology often allow a firm diagnosis. HRCT can be very helpful in suggesting the diagnosis and may show abnormalities when the chest radiograph is normal.

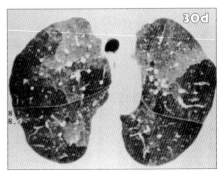

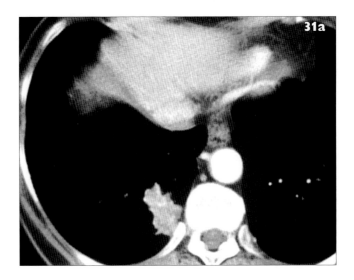

31 A 42-year-old female presented with an acute febrile illness and cough. She was diagnosed as having a right basal pneumonia and was treated with a course of antibiotics. Despite complete resolution of her symptoms, a radiographic abnormality persisted within the right lower zone for 6 months. There was a history of recurrent chest infections. She was a nonsmoker. Clinical examination was unremarkable. There was no cyanosis or clubbing. The heart and breath sounds were normal. Full blood count and biochemistry were normal. The ESR was not elevated. Other laboratory tests were also unremarkable. Due to the persisting radiographic abnormality, a CT was performed with intravenous contrast enhancement (31a).

What is the most likely diagnosis?

31: Answer

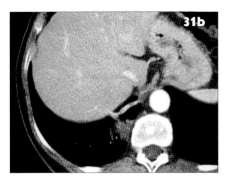 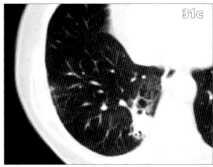

31 CT of the chest shows a 2.5 × 3.0 cm lesion in the medial aspect of the right lower lobe, abutting the pleural surface. The high attenuation foci represent contrast-enhanced vessels. A single artery is seen arising directly from the lower thoracic aorta (**31a**), and its course can be traced into the opacity within the right lower lobe (**31b**). The adjacent lung shows areas of decreased lung attenuation and cystic change (**31c**). The left lung was normal.

The diagnosis is pulmonary sequestration. The condition has been described as nonfunctional lung tissue that is not in normal continuity with the airways and has a systemic blood supply. Intra-lobar sequestrations, which share the pleura of the affected lung lobes, account for approximately three-quarters of cases. The rest are extra-lobar within a separate pleural envelope. Intra-lobar sequestration commonly presents in the second to third decade with recurrent chest infections. The condition is very rare in infants, and may be infrequently associated with congenital abnormalities such as oesophagobronchial diverticula, diaphragmatic hernias, skeletal, cardio-vascular, and renal abnormalities. Pathologically, intra-lobar sequestration is characterized by chronic inflammation, fibrosis, vascular sclerosis, and cystic change.

On chest radiography, an uncomplicated sequestrated segment may present as an area of consolidation or a mass within the lower lobe. Aerated sequestrated segments may be radiographically cryptic. Cavitation is not an unusual finding, and cystic spaces which contain fluid levels may be seen. CT is diagnostic when the anomalous artery is demonstrated, and this can be demonstrated in the majority of cases with the aid of multiplanar reformatted images. The artery appears as a tubular enhancing structure between the descending aorta and the sequestrated segment. Emphysema-like changes and modelling abnormality of the surrounding lung are common on CT. Angiography may be required to characterize the venous drainage of the seque-stration. The majority of intra-lobar sequestrations have a venous drainage via the pulmonary veins (95%). Extra-lobar sequestration usually has a systemic drainage (80%) via the azygos or hemiazygos veins. Treatment is usually surgical resection with segmentectomy or lobectomy. There have been rare reports of adenocarcinoma or squamous cell carcinoma arising within a sequestrated segment.

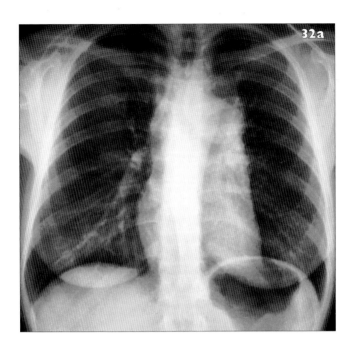

32a

32 A 42-year-old female presented to her family doctor with night sweats and feeling unwell. There was no relevant past medical history and she was normally fit and worked as a receptionist. Routine blood tests were normal. A chest radiograph was performed (32a).
i. What are the findings?
ii. How should these be confirmed?
iii. What is the differential diagnosis?

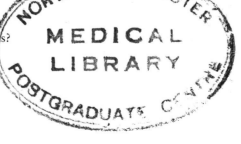

32: Answer

32 i. The radiograph shows widening of the superior mediastinum (32a). The outlines of the descending aorta and left hilum are not obscured and the hilar structures can still be identified. The lungs are clear and the heart size is normal. The features are those of an anterior mediastinal mass.

ii. A lateral radiograph confirms this suspicion as there is increased soft tissue attenuation in the retrosternal area (the density of the costophrenic angle region posteriorly should be the same as that of the retrocardiac region) (32b). Non-enhanced CT also shows the abnormality to be within the anterior mediastinum (32c). It is of near homogeneous soft tissue density and no areas of fat density or calcification are seen.

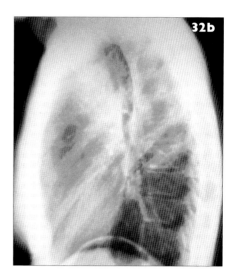

iii. The differential diagnosis of an anterior mediastinal mass includes lymphoma, germ cell tumour, thymic tumour, lymphadenopathy, or a retrosternal thyroid (although thyroid extension into the thorax may also occur within the middle or posterior mediastinum). The mass was biopsied under ultrasound guidance and found to be a non-Hodgkin's lymphoma.

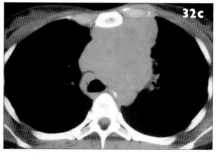

Non-Hodgkin's lymphomas are neoplasms of a specific type of lymphoreticular cell and either B-lymphocytes, T-lymphocytes, or histiocytes are involved. The commonest feature of non-Hodgkin's lymphoma on the chest radiograph is mediastinal and hilar lymphadenopathy. The anterior and paratracheal nodes are most frequently affected, whereas posterior mediastinal lymphadenopathy is rare. Hodgkin's lymphoma commonly involves more than two nodal groups, whereas one-half of the patients with non-Hodgkin's lymphoma have disease localized to a single nodal site. Identification of lymph node calcification is very rare pre-treatment, but may be seen after therapy.

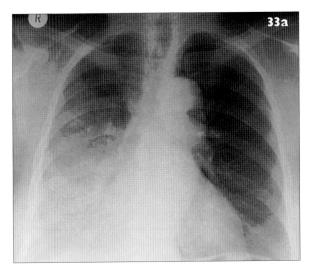

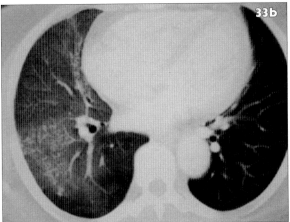

33 A 61-year-old female developed increasing breathlessness and a cough with occasional production of blood. She was a nonsmoker. The chest radiograph showed an abnormality which had persisted for 2 months despite antibiotic treatment. On examination, she looked well and was not pyrexial or obviously anaemic. Respiratory function tests revealed normal lung volumes. The chest radiograph findings (33a) prompted a bronchoscopy and biopsies were taken.

i. Describe the radiographic and CT (33b) findings.

ii. What is the likely diagnosis?

33 i. The chest radiograph shows ill-defined consolidation and ground-glass opacity within the right mid and lower zones (**33a**). The left lung is clear. The appearances are confirmed on CT, which shows that the increased density involves both the right lower and right middle lobes (**33b**). Several ill-defined nodules are superimposed on the increased density in the right lower lobe.

ii. The diagnosis of bronchioloalveolar cell carcinoma (BAC) was made on bronchoscopic biopsy. The diagnosis of BAC is often delayed. This is partly because over 50% of cases are asymptomatic at presentation and because of misdiagnosis as other conditions, usually pneumonia. BAC is a subtype of adenocarcinoma and represents 2–10% of all lung cancers. The tumour spreads locally using the lung structure as a stroma (so-called 'lepidic' growth). Radiographically there are three characteristic appearances:

- Single pulmonary nodule. This form has the best prognosis (70% successful surgical resection) and is the commonest type. On chest radiography it appears as a solitary nodule or mass, frequently subpleural with a pleural tag. This sign is not specific however, also being seen with benign scars, granulomas, and adeno-carcinoma. Although a solitary nodule may progress to diffuse disease (see below), such progression is unusual. Of note, BAC is a cause of a false-negative result on PET scanning.
- An area of consolidation. This is the second commonest manifestation and may be associated with copious mucus production (bronchorrhoea) resulting in expansion of a lobe and bulging fissures. Additional, discrete nodules in the same or different lobes are seen in over 50% of cases and are associated with a poorer prognosis.
- Multiple nodules. This form has the worst prognosis and its appearance is similar to that of metastatic disease from an extrathoracic primary tumour.

The CT appearances are characterized by air bronchograms and bubble-like areas of low attenuation within areas of consolidation. These are due to patent small airways or cystic areas within the nodule. Spiculation is common in the focal form, due to a desmoplastic response. The diffuse form may appear as multiple, poorly defined areas of ground-glass attenuation (as in this case) or consolidation. Thickened interlobular septa may be seen giving a 'crazy-paving' type appearance. Pleural effusion and hilar or mediastinal lymphadenopathy may also be seen.

BAC usually contains some areas of ground-glass attenuation at thin-section CT. When combined with a bubble-like low attenuation and persistence or progression over >6–8 weeks, the findings should help distinguish the solitary form from pulmonary eosinophilia, lymphoma, and haemorrhagic nodules. The consolidative form needs to be distinguished from pneumonia, aspiration, and pulmonary oedema. BAC may be suggested by a combination of clinical history, the presence of any additional satellite nodules, and its peripheral distribution. The multinodular form should be differentiated from fungal infection, granulomatous disease (e.g. Wegener's granulomatosis and TB), lymphoma, and metastatic carcinoma.

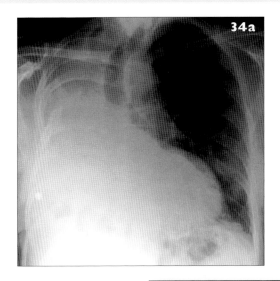

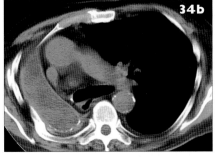

34 A 75-year-old male had a procedure performed 2 years previously. The chest radiograph and CT are shown (**34a, b**).
i. What was the procedure?
ii. What was the likely reason?

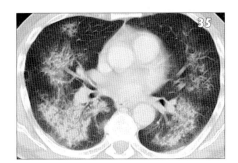

35 A 71-year-old male presented with a history of nonproductive cough, weight loss, fatigue, and shortness of breath. The radiographs (not shown) had initially shown bilateral airspace consolidation which had not improved over the course of 4 weeks, despite broad spectrum antibiotics.
i. What does the CT (**35**) show?
ii. What is the differential diagnosis?

34, 35: Answers

34 i. The patient has had a right pneumonectomy.

ii. The reason for the procedure was most probably lung cancer. The radiograph and CT show the typical appearances, with marked loss of volume within the right hemithorax (note the tracheal deviation) (**34a, b**). The ribs also appear abnormal on the right due to healing post-resection. The pneumonectomy space gradually becomes filled with fluid over the course of several weeks post-operatively (note the fluid attenuation on CT). The CT also demonstrates calcification of the parietal pleura.

35 i. The CT shows bilateral consolidation with air bronchograms, with a perihilar distribution in the lower lobes (**35**). Indistinctly marginated areas of opacification are also seen in the right middle lobe and lingula.

ii. The differential diagnosis for bilateral persisting areas of consolidation would include bronchioloalveolar cell carcinoma, organizing pneumonia, eosinophilic pneumonia, pulmonary lymphoma, or atypical infections if the patient is immuno-compromised. A bronchoscopy was performed with bronchoalveolar lavage and transbronchial biopsy. *Pneumocystis carinii* organisms were identified on light microscopy and subsequently the patient was found to be HIV-positive.

The human immunodeficiency virus is a retrovirus responsible for AIDS which affects cell-mediated immunity by attaching to the CD4 surface glycoprotein of helper T-lymphocytes. *Pneumocystis carinii* pneumonia (PCP) is the commonest infection in the developed world when the CD4 count is <0.2×10^9/l (200 lymphocytes/mm^3). The organism used to be responsible for death due to respiratory failure in a significant proportion of patients before the introduction of effective prophylaxis.

The radiographic appearances of PCP are of a bilateral, perihilar fine opacification which progresses to consolidation and sometimes a coarse reticular pattern if the infection persists. Thickened interlobular septa are common. However, the chest radiograph may be normal. HRCT is more sensitive and may show ground-glass opacity not appreciated on the radiograph. Pneumatoceles are also common and are present on CT in about one-third of cases. Atypical findings described in PCP include lobar consolidation mimicking a pyogenic pneumonia, nodules with or without cavitation, miliary nodules, pleural effusions, and mediastinal and hilar lymphadenopathy.

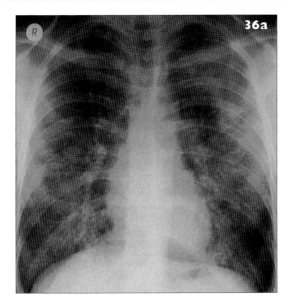

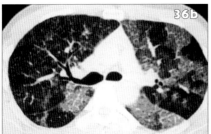
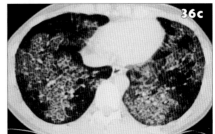

36 A 51-year-old male presented with mild increasing shortness of breath over several months after an abnormality was picked up on a pre-operative chest radiograph. He was a heavy smoker and had had hepatitis A in the past. On examination, he was not clubbed and had normal breath sounds. He had an elevated ESR but otherwise blood tests were unremarkable. Lung function tests showed a reduced DL_{CO} (48% of predicted).

i. What do the radiograph (36a) and HRCT (36b, c) show?

ii. How is this condition treated?

36: Answer

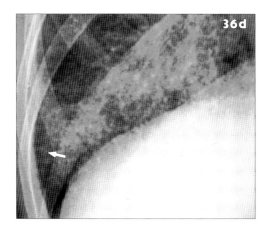

36 i. The radiograph shows patchy, bilateral areas of airspace opacification with septal lines at the bases (36d, arrow). HRCT demonstrates patchy, ground-glass opacity, sharply demarcated from surrounding normal lung, creating a 'geographic' pattern (36b, c). Smooth thickening of intralobular structures and interlobular septa is visible within areas of ground-glass opacification, often in polygonal shapes and hence the term 'crazy paving' pattern. The diagnosis is pulmonary alveolar proteinosis and the interstitial abnormality has been shown to be due to septal oedema and accumulation of phospholipids in the interlobular septa. The alveoli are filled with lipoproteinaceous material. The differential diagnosis includes opportunistic infection such as *Pneumocystis carinii* pneumonia (PCP) or cytomegalovirus (CMV) and bronchioloalveolar cell carcinoma.

ii. Treatment is by bronchoalveolar lavage; in some patients this results in remission of the disease, but others require repeated treatments.

Pulmonary alveolar proteinosis is a rare disease of unknown aetiology, characterized by filling of alveolar spaces with PAS-positive lipoproteinaceous material. Two forms have been described: 'primary' with no identifiable cause, and 'secondary' which is associated with haematological conditions, such as lymphoma or leukaemia, or exposure to inhaled dust or fumes. The pathogenesis is believed to involve excessive secretion and/or disrupted clearance of surfactant by alveolar macrophages. The condition may be complicated by infection by opportunistic organisms due to macrophage impairment. Common organisms include *Nocardia* sp., *Mycobacterium tuberculosis*, nontuberculous mycobacteria, and cryptococcus.

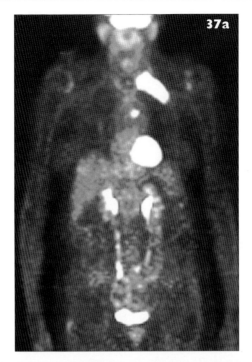

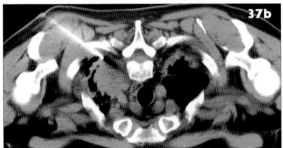

37 A 72-year-old female presented with left shoulder pain and a left-sided Horner's syndrome (miosis, enophthalmos, and ptosis). She had been a smoker in the past. On examination, she was underweight but not clubbed. There were no palpable lymph nodes.

i. What is the examination in **37a** and what does it show?

ii. What subsequent procedure is shown (**37b**)?

37: Answer

37 i. 37a shows an image from a [^{18}F]-fluorodeoxyglucose (FDG) positron emission tomography (PET) study. There is increased uptake of tracer at the left apex of the lung (37c, large arrow) and within a mediastinal lymph node (small arrow). Note the normal uptake of tracer in the posterior fossa and myocardium and excretion by the kidneys into the bladder. FDG is a glucose analogue (with ^{18}F substituted for a hydroxy group) which becomes trapped in tumour cells after phosphorylation. It is a marker of glucose metabolism and may show increased activity in other nonmalignant processes such as infection. However, it is extremely useful in staging of malignancies such as lung cancer, to show mediastinal lymph nodes involved by tumour, as in this patient, and distant metastases.

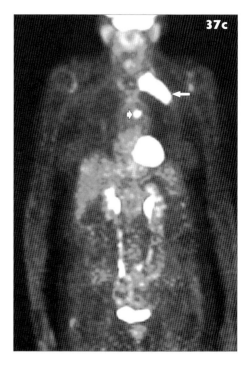

ii. 37b shows an image from a CT-guided biopsy of the left apical or superior sulcus mass. The patient is lying prone and the biopsy needle is seen entering the mass obliquely (to avoid bony structures) via a posterior approach. Histology showed a squamous cell carcinoma.

Superior sulcus tumours are also known as Pancoast's tumours when there are the clinical features of an ipsilateral Horner's syndrome and pain in the arm or shoulder due to local invasion of the adjacent brachial plexus and sympathetic chain. Pain may also be due to local destruction of bone by tumour. MRI may be useful to show involvement of the adjacent brachial plexus, subclavian vessels, and bone marrow.

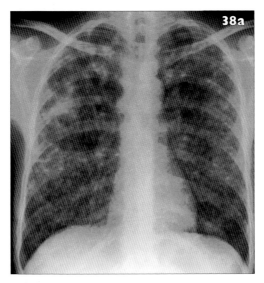

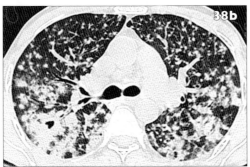

38 A 43-year-old male waiter presented with increasing shortness of breath, fevers, and lethargy. He was normally fit and well apart from using inhalers for asthma. He had had a recent exacerbation of asthma requiring hospital admission and was still taking oral corticosteroids. He had lived in India for the first 20 years of his life and had immigrated to London. He had a large, extended family and made frequent trips back to the Indian subcontinent, the last being 1 month previously.

His chest radiograph and HRCT are shown (38a, b) .

i. What are the findings?

ii. What is the likely diagnosis?

38: Answer

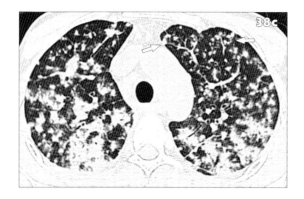

38 i. The chest radiograph shows bilateral airspace opacification, which is becoming confluent in some areas such as the right mid and upper zone (38a). There are also widespread, nodular opacities bilaterally. No definite areas of cavitation are seen on the radiograph, but a cavitating area is clearly seen within the posterior segment of the right upper lobe on the HRCT (performed 24 hours later, 38b). Also note the nodular appearance demonstrated on the HRCT: some of the larger nodules represent airspaces filled with exudate, others reflect secretions in the small airways 'tree-in-bud pattern' (38c, arrows).

ii. Acid-fast bacilli were isolated from sputum and a diagnosis of tuberculous bronchopneumonia was made.

Tuberculous bronchopneumonia is a form of reactivation TB and may be encountered in immunocompromised hosts. The process may involve a lobe or all the lungs, as in this case. Cavitation is frequent and may be more easily appreciated with CT, because of the lack of superimposed structures. Seeding of the bronchial tree occurs, particularly with cavitation, giving rise to the 'tree-in-bud' appearance which spreads to other parts of the lungs. Widespread bronchopneumonia usually results from a breakdown in host immunity and may involve regions of the lung not usually affected by TB, such as the anterior part of the upper lobes and the middle lobe.

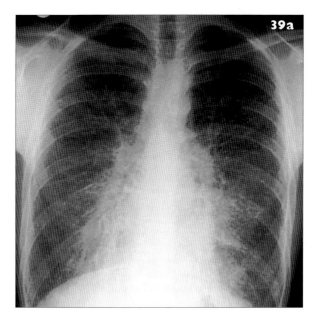

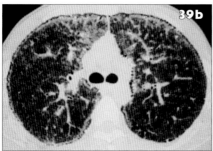

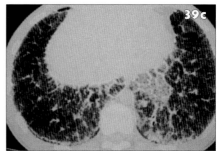

39 A 17-year-old male was referred with a history of increased shortness of breath on exertion. He had had a past medical history of asthma since the age of 6 years old. He smoked 5–6 cigarettes a day. On examination, he was thin but otherwise well with no clubbing, lymphadenopathy, or cyanosis. There were minimal bilateral basal crackles on auscultation. Sweat test, serum ACE, full blood count, and urea and electrolytes were normal. Lung function tests showed FEV_1 and FVC at 85% of predicted normal values with a normal flow-volume loop.

i. What do the chest radiograph (39a) and HRCT (39b, c) show?

ii. What might be the (rare!) diagnosis?

39: Answer

39 i. The chest radiograph shows diffuse micronodular shadowing with preservation of lung volume. The cardiac borders are obscured. The HRCT scans show multiple small nodules with a subpleural distribution and multiple small subpleural cysts (**39b, c**). There are a few thickened interlobular septa.

ii. The diagnosis is alveolar microlithiasis, a rare cause of miliary nodules (see Question 85). The aetiology and pathogenesis are unknown. Histopathological appearances show rounded, concentrically laminated psammoma-like bodies called calcospherites of between 150 and 200 μm which fill the alveoli. Small bullae may be seen. Although it is a very rare disease, it

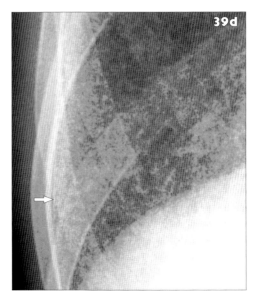

has characteristic radiographic appearances. Fine, sand-like nodular calcific deposits are demonstrated with a mid- to lower-zone predominance on the chest radiograph. The heart and diaphragmatic contours may be obscured. Pleural calcification and ground-glass opacity have also been described. The 'black stripe' sign is characteristic and describes the pleura appearing black by comparison with the adjacent ribs and finely calcified lung parenchyma (**39d**, arrow).

The HRCT demonstrates micronodular calcific densities in a fairly random distribution, but most numerous in the lower lobes. Multiple thin-walled small subpleural cysts are also particularly well shown along the mediastinal and chest wall pleural interface, and explain the high incidence of pneumothorax in the condition. There may also be thickened interlobular septa and peribronchovascular interstitium.

An open lung biopsy was performed to secure the diagnosis. The prognosis varies but respiratory failure eventually develops in virtually all patients.

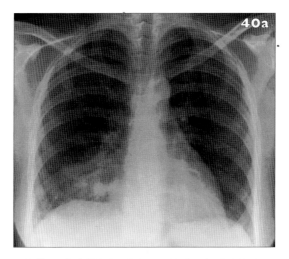

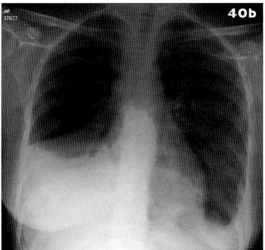

40 A 31-year-old female presented with a cough which had persisted despite antibiotic treatment. Two radiographs are shown which were obtained 2 months apart (40a, b). On direct questioning she revealed that she had had some difficulty swallowing recently.

i. What do the radiographs show?

ii. What radiological investigation should be performed next?

40: Answer

40 i. The initial chest radiograph shows patchy consolidation which is obscuring the right heart border,
consistent with right middle lobe consolidation (40a). The
subsequent radiograph shows increased opacity in the right
lower zone, consistent with a combination of right lower
lobe and right middle lobe collapse (both the right heart
border and right hemidiaphragm contour are obscured)
(40b). In addition, the left hemidiaphragm is obscured and
there is blunting of the left costophrenic angle, suggestive
of left lower lobe consolidation and a small pleural effusion. The distribution of abnormalities in the dependent
areas and the presence of different lobes being affected
raises the possibility of repeated episodes of aspiration.
ii. A barium swallow was performed because of these
findings and her difficulty in swallowing (40c, d). The
lateral view of the upper oesophagus shows barium spilling
over into the trachea (40c, arrow) and views of the lung
bases confirm bilateral aspirated barium within the
bronchial tree. Subsequently, she was found to have a
neurological cause for her aspiration, a cerebellar tumour.

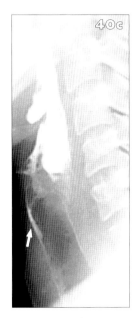

The extent of radiographic abnormality in
aspiration depends on the volume and chemical
and physical properties of the aspirated liquid.
Large amounts of gastric secretions may be
aspirated in certain clinical scenarios (e.g. during
states of decreased conciousness), giving rise to
widespread bilateral airspace opacification
similar to pulmonary oedema or permeability
oedema due to acute respiratory distress
syndrome (ARDS). In uncomplicated cases, the
findings usually resolve over a period of several
days. However, complications such as ARDS,

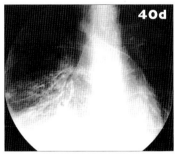

bacterial pneumonia, or pulmonary embolus may occur. When there is aspiration of
smaller volumes of oropharyngeal contents, the appearance may resemble a bacterial
pneumonia, although the distribution tends to involve the dependent portion of the
lungs and to be accompanied by a degree of atelectasis. In cases where there is
repeated aspiration, areas of atelectasis and consolidation may come and go in
different anatomical sites on serial radiographs over a period of months or years.
Conditions that predispose to aspiration include chronic debilitating illness,
oropharyngeal or airway instrumentation, unconscious or decreased conscious states,
and disorders affecting swallowing (e.g. achalasia and neuromuscular disease).

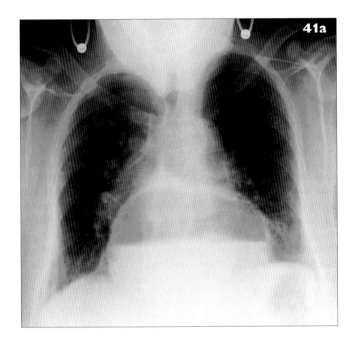

41 A 75-year-old female presented with symptoms of chest pain. On examination, she was well, apyrexial, and not clubbed. Her full blood count showed a mild iron deficiency anaemia. All other investigations (including an ECG) were normal.

What does the chest radiograph show (41a)?

45: Answer

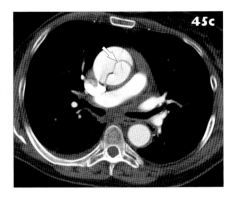

45 i. The chest radiograph, even allowing for the AP projection, shows widening of the mediastinum, particularly in the region of the ascending thoracic aorta (45a). The trachea is slightly deviated to the right. He had a blood pressure of 150/90 mmHg (20/12 kPa) in his right arm and 130/70 mmHg (17.3/9.3 kPa) in his left arm. A CT was performed which shows a fine, linear structure (45c, arrow) consistent with an intimal flap involving the ascending thoracic aorta, which is slightly dilated. Note also the increased soft tissue attenuation in the mediastinum (representing haematoma) and the small right pleural effusion. The descending aorta is not involved. The diagnosis is a Type A thoracic aortic dissection.

ii. The differentiation of Type A (involving the ascending thoracic aorta) and Type B (confined to the descending thoracic aorta irrespective of the site of primary intimal tear) is important for patient management. Type A dissections may involve the aortic root and aortic valve, resulting in aortic regurgitation (also diagnosed in this case, the clinical sign being an early diastolic murmur), may rupture into the pericardium resulting in haemopericardium and cardiac tamponade or may involve the coronary arteries or the major arteries arising from the aortic arch. The outcome of patients with Type A dissection is significantly improved when surgery is performed, whereas patients with Type B dissection are often first treated medically, reserving surgery for persisting or progressive symptoms.

The radiographic signs include widening of the mediastinum due to increased diameter of the ascending or descending aorta or mediastinal haematoma, a wide or indistinct aortic knuckle, an apical cap (extra-pleural blood), pleural effusion (usually on the left), and tracheal shift. However, a portable AP radiograph is often obtained as the patient is unwell, and these signs may be difficult to distinguish confidently from the apparent widening that occurs on an AP projection in normal cases. Progressive widening on serial studies is more specific for the diagnosis.

CT is much more sensitive and specific than radiography for aortic dissection, typically demonstrating the true and false lumens, separated by the curvilinear intimal flap. The false lumen may have decreased contrast enhancement, due to either reduced flow or thrombus. Multiplanar reconstructions may aid assessment of extension of the dissection into the major arteries originating from the aortic arch, or the renal and mesenteric arteries in a Type B dissection.

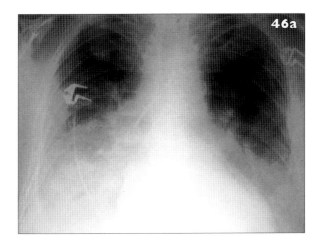

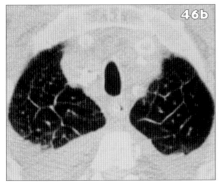

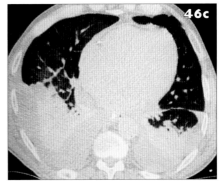

46 A 52-year-old male was admitted with unstable angina and pulmonary oedema. He subsequently deteriorated, requiring inotropic support and the insertion of an intra-aortic balloon pump. Amiodarone was started to control cardiac arrythmias. He subsequently underwent a cardiac angiogram which demonstrated complete occlusion of his right coronary artery and 60% stenosis of the left anterior descending coronary artery. A balloon dilatation and stenting of the left anterior descending artery were successfully performed. His blood pressure was 150/80 mmHg (20/10.7 kPa), with a heart rate of 80 beats per minute. He was apyrexial and had no pulses below his femorals. The heart sounds were inaudible and he had decreased air entry at both lung bases. A 4 cm liver edge was palpable. Full blood count was normal. He had moderate renal impairment and mildly deranged liver function tests.

What do the radiograph (46a) and CT (46b, c) show?

46: Answer

46 A mobile AP erect radiograph, taken shortly after admission to the intensive care unit, shows a tracheostomy tube and a left internal jugular intravenous catheter (**46a**). The coronary artery stent is just visible. There is ground-glass opacification in the mid zones, and more confluent dense opacification in the lower zones obscuring both hemidiaphragms. There is peribronchial cuffing and increase in size of the upper lobe vessels. The radiographic features are consistent with pulmonary oedema but an HRCT was performed to exclude additional pathology that would explain his ventilator-dependency. The HRCT show areas of ground-glass attenuation and smooth thickening of interlobular septa, most apparent at the apices (**46b, c**). There is also peribronchovascular thickening. There are bilateral pleural effusions and bilateral lower lobe collapse. The HRCT features are consistent with hydrostatic pulmonary oedema.

Hydrostatic pulmonary oedema can be defined as an abnormal increase in extravascular water, secondary to elevated pressures in the pulmonary circulation as in congestive cardiac failure or intravascular volume overload. The radiographic features of hydrostatic pulmonary oedema are: septal lines (Kerley A and B lines), ground-glass opacification which obscures vessels, peribronchial cuffing representing interstitial oedema, increase in size of the upper lobe vessels (a common early sign of left heart failure), consolidation, and pleural effusions. In the setting of the current clinical scenario, the features which sometimes allow distinction from acute respiratory distress syndrome (ARDS) are the redistribution of pulmonary blood flow to the upper lobes, the distribution of pulmonary oedema, and the width of the vascular pedicle (although the latter is difficult to assess accurately on a single portable AP radiograph). Nevertheless, in most cases the distinction between ARDS and hydrostatic pulmonary oedema on the basis of the chest radiographic findings alone is difficult or impossible.

The typical HRCT features of hydrostatic pulmonary oedema are demonstrated in the current case, and consist of bilateral thickening of the interlobular septa and peribronchovascular intersitium and ground-glass opacities or consolidation. Usually, but by no means invariably, the ground-glass opacity has a predominantly gravitational or central distribution. The classification of pulmonary oedema into either cardiogenic or noncardiogenic oedema may be oversimplistic as cardiogenic pulmonary oedema is not necessarily purely hydrostatic, in that capillary endothelium damage may occur resulting in permeability oedema; permeability oedema can occur without diffuse alveolar damage (DAD), thus causing different radiographic appearances, e.g. interleukin-2 administration and hantavirus pulmonary syndrome. The classification system which has recently been advocated recognizes four categories: (1) hydrostatic oedema; (2) permeability oedema caused by DAD; (3) permeability oedema without DAD; and (4) mixed hydrostatic and permeability oedema.

47 A 49-year-old female presented with a persistent cough and her family doctor referred her for a chest radiograph (47a). On examination, she was well, with no lymphadenopathy or clubbing. Her full blood count, urea and electolytes, and liver function tests were all normal.
i. What are the radiographic findings?
ii. What does the CT show (47b)?

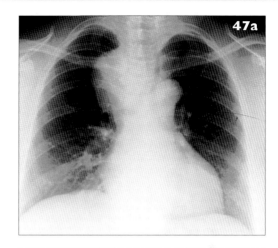

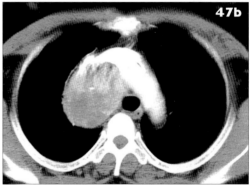

48 A 45-year-old male presented to his family doctor with a persistent productive cough. He had been treated in the past for a chest condition. The doctor requested a chest radiograph (48).
i. What are the findings?
ii. What is a differential diagnosis?

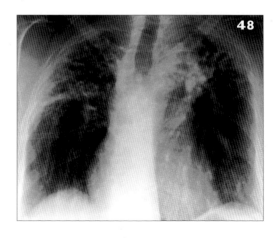

47 i. The chest radiograph shows a large superior mediastinal mass which is deviating the trachea to the left, but not causing any narrowing of the tracheal lumen (**47a**). The lateral edge of the mass is seen to be well defined and extends superiorly above the right clavicle. This sign is helpful in placing the mass as within the middle or posterior mediastinum, as anterior mediastinal mass lateral borders lose their definition above the clavicles due to the oblique orientation of the thoracic inlet in a sagittal plane (i.e. the thoracic inlet is lower anteriorly than posteriorly and so anterior mediastinal masses no longer form a silhouette with aerated lung above the clavicles).

ii. The CT demonstrates the mass to the right of the trachea, and displacing the superior vena cava anteriorly and laterally (**47b**). The calibre of the trachea is normal. The mass has slightly heterogeneous contrast opacification and contains a small fleck of calcification centrally. The mass was surgically removed and found to be a benign thyroid goitre.

The case demonstrates the typical radiographic appearances of an intrathoracic goitre. A well-defined border and tracheal displacement (or narrowing) are very common. The goitre may be predominantly anterior, lateral (as in this case), or posterior to the trachea. Calcification is common in benign goitres, but also may occur in malignant thyroid tumours. Therefore, definitive distinction of benign from malignant thyroid mass is difficult with CT, unless there is evidence of either local or distant disease spread. Another useful sign illustrated by this case is enhancement of some parts of the mass to a greater degree by comparison with adjacent muscle, due to avid uptake of iodine by thyroid tissue. In most cases, contiguous extension of intrathoracic goitres from the thyroid gland in the neck is readily apparent on CT. However, in some cases there is only a thin fibrous band between the intrathoracic mass and the thyroid gland, and in such cases the features described above may be helpful in suggesting the correct diagnosis.

48 i. The chest radiograph shows marked bilateral upper lobe fibrosis with elevation of both hila, increased coarse linear opacification within both upper lobes, and compensatory hyperinflation in the lower lobes (**48**). Within the upper zones bilaterally, there are ring shadows caused by traction bronchiectasis. Mediastinal lymph node calcification is also noted.

ii. The differential diagnosis for bilateral upper lobe fibrosis includes previous TB, pulmonary sarcoidosis, previous radiotherapy, and ankylosing spondylitis. In this case, the patient had been treated for sarcoidosis in the past.

In 5–25% of patients with pulmonary sarcoidosis, the initial radiograph may show severe fibrosis. In a further 10–15% of cases, marked fibrosis occurs in patients who present with either a normal radiograph, hilar adenopathy alone, or with parenchymal involvement. The fibrosis usually takes several years to develop. It is almost always confined to the upper and mid zones, and on CT or a lateral radiograph, the first areas to be affected are usually the posterior parts of the upper lobes. Occasionally, the fibrosis may be so severe that it mimics the progessive massive fibrosis seen in coal worker's pneumoconiosis. Cor pulmonale may complicate fibrotic sarcoidosis, as shown radiographically by dilatation of central pulmonary arteries.

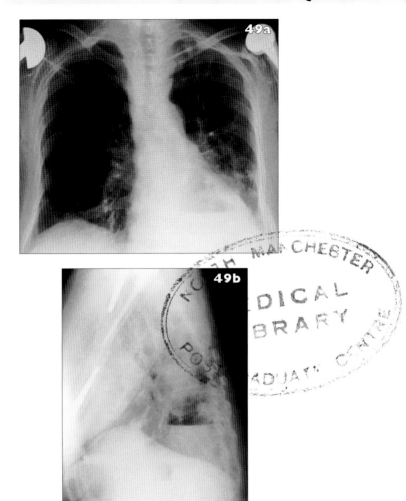

49 A 58-year-old female presented with a cough, fever, and feeling unwell and feverish for a couple of weeks. She had a past history of rheumatoid arthritis and was on long-term corticosteroid therapy. On examination, she had evidence of rheumatoid arthritis affecting her hands and feet. She was pyrexial and had reduced breath sounds and a dull percussion note at the left base. She also had a raised white cell count, CRP, and ESR. A chest radiograph (PA and left lateral) was performed (49a, b).
i. What are the radiological findings?
ii. What is a likely diagnosis?

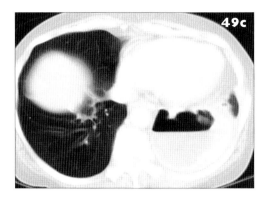

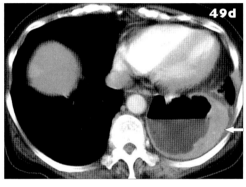

49 i. The PA and lateral radiographs show an air–fluid level in the left lower zone posteriorly, resembling a hiatus hernia but, in the clinical context, likely to represent either a large lung abscess or empyema (with bronchopleural fistula) (**49a, b**). Note the bilateral shoulder replacements. The abnormality was confirmed to be intrapulmonary on CT (**49c**) since peripheral enhancing lung was demonstrated (**49d**, arrow).

ii. The diagnosis is a large pulmonary abscess due to anaerobic bacterial infection, and the abscess was drained at thoracotomy. Other radiological differential diagnoses include a large cavitating rheumatoid nodule, TB, and a cavitating bronchogenic carcinoma.

Cavitation with consolidation usually suggests fungal or bacterial infection. The common organisms to consider are *Staphylococcus aureus*, *Klebsiella* sp., *Mycobacterium tuberculosis*, and anaerobic bacteria. In large, solitary abscesses without underlying lung disease, aspiration of gastric contents or underlying host immune impairment should be considered as contributing or causative factors.

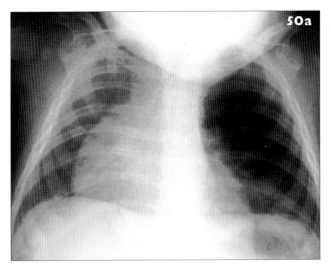

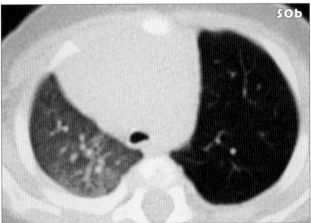

50 A 6-month-old well male presented in the neonatal period with tachypnoea. He was born at 42 weeks gestation with a satisfactory Apgar score. There was a history of premature rupture of membranes 12 days prior to delivery and he was treated on the Special Care Baby Unit for possible infection (blood cultures were subsequently negative). On examination, he appeared well (50th centile for height and weight). There were reduced breath sounds in the left upper zone posteriorly. Other systems were unremarkable.

What do the chest radiograph and CT show (50a, b) ?

50: Answer

50 The chest radiograph shows hyperinflation of the left lung with mediastinal shift to the right and loss of volume of the right lung (**50a**). The CT demonstrates increased transradiancy and increased volume of the left upper lobe (**50b**). The trachea appears of normal calibre. The findings are consistent with congenital lobar emphysema (CLE).

CLE refers to the progressive overdistension of one or more pulmonary lobes, resulting in compression of the adjacent normal lung. One-half of the cases present with severe respiratory distress within the first 1–2 days post-delivery and require early surgery. The remaining patients develop symptoms between 1 and 4 months, although asymptomatic forms have been reported in late childhood or even adulthood. The pathogenesis of CLE is obscure; in some cases there may be a bronchial cartilage deficiency or immaturity, or an intrinsic obstruction such as a mucous plug or web. Extrinsic causes include vascular rings and slings or bronchogenic cysts. However, in 50% of cases the cause remains unknown. Ten to fifteen percent are associated with congenital heart disease such as a patent ductus arteriosus or ventricular septal defect. The incidence of CLE is highest in Caucasian males with a male to female ratio of 3:1. The left upper lobe is most commonly affected, followed by the right middle lobe and right upper lobe, with the lower lobes being rarely affected.

Initial radiographs may show an opaque lobe or hemithorax due to delayed clearance of pulmonary fluid (which may mimic a mass lesion). Typically, the fluid clears to reveal an underlying hyperlucent expanded lobe. Vascular markings can be seen in the affected lobe which helps to differentiate CLE from a tension pneumothorax, congenital lung cyst, or cystic adenomatoid malformation. CT is of value in demonstrating any causative pathology (such as vascular rings), the degree of overinflation, and excluding bronchial atresia. VQ scanning may be used to measure regional lung function and monitor progress in conjunction with the chest radiograph. Resection of the affected lobe may be necessary, but in many cases the treatment is expectant.

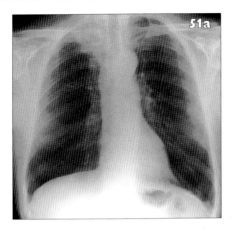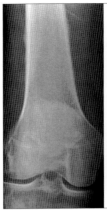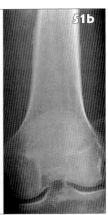

51 A 77-year-old male presented with cough, weight loss, and pains in his lower limbs. He was an ex-smoker. Radiographs of his chest and distal femurs are shown (51a, b).
What is the unifying diagnosis?

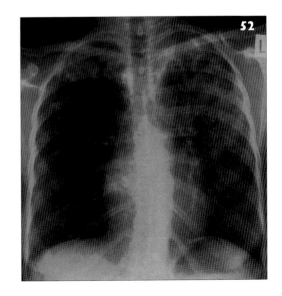

52 A 67-year-old female from the Indian subcontinent presented with a productive cough, fever, and weight loss. She was previously well but had a history of pulmonary tuberculosis (TB) some 15 years previously. On examination, she was thin with coarse crepitations on auscultation at the left mid zone. Her radiograph is shown (52).
i. What are the radiographic findings and the likely diagnosis?
ii. Are there any immediate precautions which should be taken?

51, 52: Answers

51 The chest radiograph shows abnormal density at the right apex (51a). There is no definite bone destruction. No other lesions are demonstrated. There is widening of the right paratracheal region, indicating lymphadenopathy. No hilar lymphadenopathy is demonstrated. The radiographs of the distal femurs show a bilateral periosteal reaction (51c, arrows). The unifying diagnosis is a right superior sulcus lung cancer (or Pancoast's tumour) with hypertrophic pulmonary osteoarthropathy (HPOA).

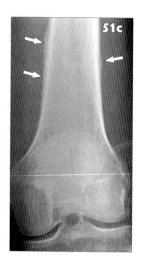

The imaging features of superior sulcus tumours are discussed in Question 37. The clinical features of HPOA include finger clubbing and painful, swollen joints. The pulmonary causes of the condition include bronchogenic carcinoma, abscess, bronchiectasis, metastases, cystic fibrosis, and malignant mesothelioma. Malignant causes such as bronchogenic carcinoma and mesothelioma most frequently result in radiographic abnormalities. Periosteal and endosteal new bone formation are seen most commonly in the bones of the lower leg and forearm, with subsequent involvement of the hands and feet. The epiphyseal regions are usually spared and the periosteal new bone usually affects the metaphysis and diaphysis. There may be dramatic resolution of symptoms and signs following resection of the primary lesion.

52 i. The radiograph shows bilateral upper lobe volume loss consistent with scarring from previous TB (52). There is also confluent right upper-zone and left mid- and upper-zone consolidation and the suggestion of cavitation in the left upper zone. The findings are highly suspicious of reactivation TB.
ii. Cavitatory disease is highly infectious for close contacts, so immediate infective precautions should be followed on the basis of the radiographic findings.

Thoracic tuberculous infection can be divided into primary, reactivation, and tuberculous pleurisy. Commonly, reactivation TB causes subsegmental consolidation in the early phase which becomes confluent. There is a propensity for involvement of the posterior upper lobes and the apical segments of the lower lobes. Cavitation is very common and clinically significant as it correlates well with disease activity. The demonstration of air–fluid levels may be useful to diagnose reactivation TB. However, this finding may be difficult to identify with certainty in patients with extensive fibrosis and scarring due to previous infection. Often comparison with previous radiographs is very useful in this situation, but in some cases CT may be helpful. Healing is indicated radiographically by increased definition of margins of consolidation and fibrosis. Other manifestations of reactivation TB include tuberculous lobar pneumonia, endobronchial TB, tuberculoma formation, and miliary TB (which may occur in either primary or reactivation TB).

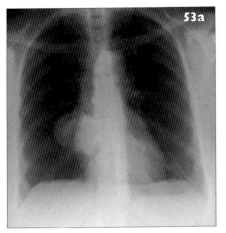

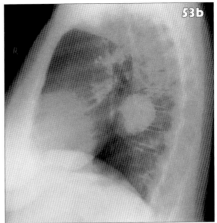

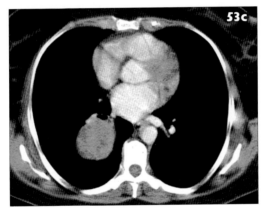

53 A 24-year-old female medical student presented with a sudden onset of haemoptysis. She had no relevant past medical history and was normally fit and well. Full blood count and urea and electrolytes were normal. Chest radiographs (53a, b) and a CT scan (53c) were obtained.
i. What are the findings?
ii. What is the differential diagnosis?

53: Answer

53 i. The chest radiographs (PA and right lateral, **53a, b**) show a large (approximately 6 cm diameter) mass, shown to be within the apical segment of the right lower lobe on CT. The CT does not demonstrate any intravenous contrast enhancement or calcification within the mass (**53c**). No definite endobronchial component is seen.

ii. Neoplastic lesions should be considered including a primary bronchial carcinoma (although the patient's age makes this unlikely), solitary pulmonary metastasis, bronchial carcinoid, an atypical hamartoma, or rare tumours such as pulmonary blastoma. Inflammatory conditions such as Wegener's granulomatosis, rheumatoid arthritis, and sarcoidosis can also present as a solitary pulmonary nodule. The nodule was resected and the diagnosis of a bronchial carcinoid was confirmed histopathologically.

Carcinoids can be divided into typical and atypical forms. Approximately 90% are typical, the rest being atypical as there are histopathological features which may be part of a spectrum between typical carcinoids and small cell lung cancer. There is a very wide age range affected from teenagers to the elderly. Most typical carcinoids arise centrally in the main, lobar, or segmental bronchi and may be either intra- or extra-luminal. They may cause bronchial obstruction and peripheral mucus impaction (bronchocele) or infection. Carcinoids are typically very vascular and may present with haemoptysis and often demonstrate avid contrast enhancement on CT. The carcinoid syndrome is extremely rare with bronchial carcinoids unless liver metastases are present. Some lesions produce ACTH and can result in Cushing's syndrome, even if the primary lesion is very small.

Carcinoids usually demonstrate uptake with radiolabelled octreotide as they contain somatostatin receptors. The lesions are usually not very metabolically active, therefore do not usually demonstrate increased activity on PET scanning.

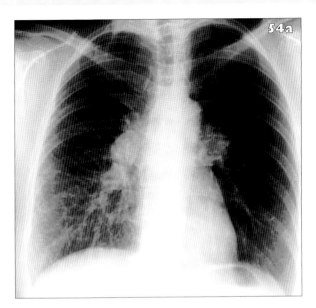

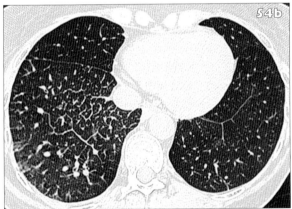

54 A 66-year-old female presented with increasing shortness of breath on exertion. She had had a left nephrectomy 1 year previously for a renal cell carcinoma. On examination, she was tachycardic (100/min) and tachypnoeic. There was no finger clubbing. The lungs were clear to auscultation. The abdomen was soft with a just palpable liver edge. No ascites was detected. Full blood count and biochemistry were normal. A chest radiograph and HRCT are shown (54a, b).

What is the diagnosis?

54: Answer

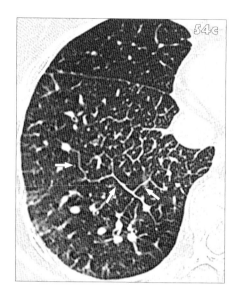

54 The chest radiograph shows prominent septal lines (Kerley B lines) in the right mid and lower zones (54a). Both hila are enlarged, but particularly the right, which also appears too dense. HRCT reveals asymmetric smooth thickening of the interlobular septa in the right lower lobe (54b).

The features are those of pulmonary lymphangitis carcinomatosa. The condition is most commonly seen with carcinoma of the breast, lung, stomach, colon, prostate, and pancreas. The term refers to the involvement of the pulmonary lymphatics with neoplastic cells. This can occur secondary to retrograde involvement of metastases to the hila or, more commonly, from haematogenous spread of tumour cells into small peripheral pulmonary arteries and then direct migration to the adjacent lymphatics. The typical radiographic finding of pulmonary lymphangitis carcinomatosa is reticulonodular shadowing, which is often diffuse and symmetrical, but may be unilateral as in this case. Accompanying mediastinal and hilar lymphadenopathy and pleural effusions are common.

HRCT is more sensitive than the radiograph in the diagnosis and detection of lymphangitis carcinomatosa. The typical HRCT findings include smooth or nodular thickening of the interlobular septa (54c, arrows), major fissures, and peribroncho-vascular interstitium. The lung architecture is preserved. The main differential diagnosis is pulmonary oedema, but in this case the unilateral nature of the disease with the enlarged hilar lymph nodes is characteristic of lymphangitis carcinomatosa.

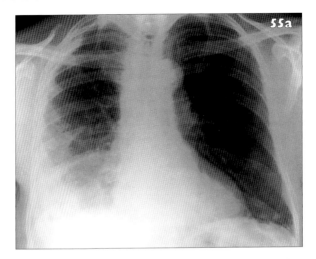

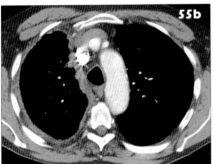 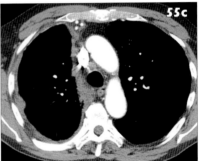

55 A 69-year-old retired electrician presented with gradual increasing shortness of breath, right-sided pleuritic chest pain, and weight loss. He had had several recent investigations including a CT of the thorax and an Abraham's needle pleural biopsy but no diagnosis had been made.

i. What do the radiograph (55a) and CT (55b, c) show?

ii. What should be done next?

55: Answer

55 i. The radiograph shows pleural thickening involving the right hemithorax with volume loss (55a). There is also widening of the right paratracheal area, which is suggestive of mediastinal lymphadenopathy. There is also increased airspace opacification at the right base and a 1.5 cm nodule within the left lower zone. No definite calcified pleural plaques are demonstrated. The CT shows pleural thickening involving the right hemithorax (55b, c). The pleural thickening is nodular, >1 cm thick, and involves the mediastinal surface (resulting in right paratracheal widening on the chest radiograph). No pleural effusion is demonstrated. The features are highly suggestive of a malignant pleural process (either malignant mesothelioma or adenocarcinoma), with a left pulmonary metastasis.

ii. The next investigation should be a repeat pleural biopsy under imaging guidance (using either ultrasound or CT) and, if this is negative, a thoracoscopic pleural biopsy. In this case, the diagnosis of malignant mesothelioma was made with an ultrasound-guided pleural biopsy.

The histological diagnosis of malignant mesothelioma may be problematic as there may be difficulty in distinguishing the process from pleural inflammation. Blind biopsy using an Abraham's needle has been found to be less accurate than radiologically-guided biopsy of pleural thickening. Histologically, malignant mesothelioma can be subdivided into epithelial, mesenchymal (either sarcomatous or fibrous), or mixed. There is a proven association with asbestos exposure and the latency between exposure and disease is 20–40 years. Although crocidolite (blue asbestos) is the most carcinogenic form, chrysotile (white asbestos) exposure accounts for the greatest number of cases as this form is in more widespread use. The prognosis is generally poor as the disease is often widespread at presentation.

The radiographic features are initially of a pleural effusion, which may not result in mediastinal shift to the contralateral side due to tumour encasement of the hemithorax. There is often progressive volume loss, and this may be readily apparent on serial chest radiographs. Pleural fluid may mask the pleural thickening and nodularity, although effusions sometimes diminish as the disease progresses. The CT features that differentiate benign pleural thickening from that due to a malignant cause include circumferential or concentric pleural thickening, pleural nodularity, and thickening >1 cm. Although these features are relatively specific, they are not 100% sensitive; therefore, absence of these findings does not completely exclude malignancy. Haematogenous or lymphatic spread of disease usually occurs relatively late; however, patients may present with mediastinal lymphadenopathy or pulmonary metastases. Local spread of disease to adjacent structures such as the chest wall and pericardium is common and may be demonstrated on CT or MRI.

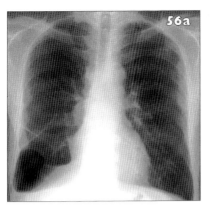

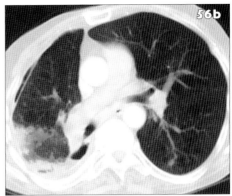

56 A 69-year-old male had a right lower lobectomy for a bronchial carcinoma. His post-operative recovery was complicated after the first week by a right-sided empyema and persistent right pneumothorax, which did not respond to percutaneous intercostal tube drainage. The chest radiograph and a section from the CT are shown (56a, b).
   Comment on the radiological findings.

57 A normally fit and healthy 35-year-old male presented with sudden onset of shortness of breath and right-sided pleuritic chest pain. He was a smoker of 20 cigarettes per day. On examination, his trachea was central but he had absent breath sounds on the right and a hyper-resonant percussion note on that side. His radiograph is shown (57).
i. What is the diagnosis?
ii. What is the the usual treatment?

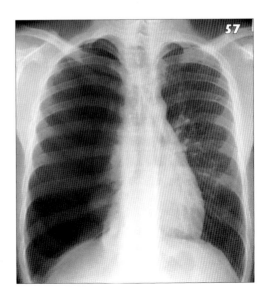

56, 57: Answers

56 The chest radiograph shows a loculated hydropneumothorax at the right base (56a). The CT shows volume loss within the right hemithorax, consistent with the patient's surgery and a small hydrothorax. There is also a tract seen which extends from bronchus intermedius to the pleural space (56c, arrow). The features are those of a bronchopleural fistula.

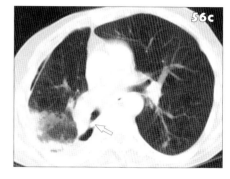

A bronchopleural fistula represents direct communication between an airway and the pleural space and is an important cause of air within the pleural space. Causes include infection (particularly necrotizing infection such as tuberculosis and anaerobes), thoracic surgery (including pneumonectomy and lobectomy), other iatrogenic causes (e.g. chest tubes, thoracocentesis), neoplasms, and radiotherapy. Post-surgical bronchopleural fistula occurs in approximately 3% of cases and is usually apparent within the first 2 post-operative weeks. The clinical features are fever, haemoptysis, and persistent air leak from the pleural drains. CT using thin sections may be helpful in defining the anatomic extent of the communicating tract. The cardinal radiographic sign of a bronchopleural fistula is new or persistent air–fluid level in the pleural space.

57 i. The radiograph shows a large right-sided pneumothorax with collapse of the underlying lung (57). In addition, there is a slight shift of the mediastinum, including trachea, to the left and flattening of the right hemidiaphragm, indicating a degree of tension. Pneumothoraces may be divided into spontaneous (when there is no precipitating trauma) and traumatic (either iatrogenic or noniatrogenic). Causes of spontaneous pneumothoraces include primary spontaneous pneumothorax and secondary pneumothoraces due to a multitude of causes such as airflow obstruction (e.g. asthma), infection (e.g. pneumatocele), infarction, neoplasia, diffuse lung disease (e.g. Langerhan's cell histiocytosis), catamenial pneumothorax (see Question 7) and inherited connective tissue disorders (e.g. Marfan's disease).

In this case, there was no obvious underlying cause. Primary spontaneous pneumothoraces occur in healthy individuals and are commoner in males, on the right, with a peak incidence between 20 and 40 years of age. There is a strong association with smoking. The incidence is approximately 10 per 100,000 population per annum.
ii. The treatment is insertion of an intercostal chest drain. The drain is connected to an underwater seal, allowing air to escape, but not to be drawn in. Occasionally, it may be necessary to use suction to allow the lung to reinflate and sometimes, in recurrent or persistent cases, chemical or surgical pleurodesis is required.

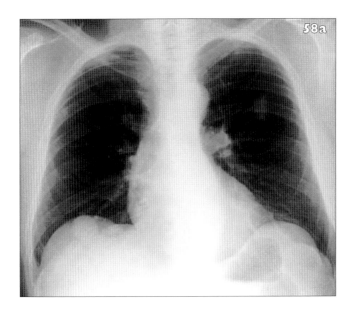

58 A 45-year-old male presented with recurrent nose bleeds. Another member of his family was being investigated for the same condition. A chest radiograph was performed (58a). There was no other relevant past medical history. Laboratory investigations were normal.
i. What does the radiograph show?
ii. What investigation should be performed next?

58: Answer

58 i. The radiograph shows multiple well-defined nodules (58b, arrows). The largest is projected behind the right hemidiaphragm, and measures approximately 2.5 cm in diameter. A supplying artery and draining vein can be seen although, as with the smaller left upper-zone nodule, these features are best appreciated on CT (58c). The features are those of multiple pulmonary arteriovenous malformations (AVM) in a patient with hereditary haemorrhagic telangiectasia (Osler–Weber–Rendu disease).

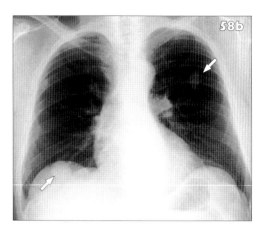

Patients with hereditary haemorrhagic telangiectasia are usually asymptomatic from pulmonary AVMs, although because of right-to-left shunting, cerebral or other systemic abscesses or infarctions may occur. The shunting may also cause hypoxia, which is more marked when the patient is erect (so-called orthodeoxia). The explanation for this phenomenon is that the lesions are more prevalent in the lower lobes and shunting is

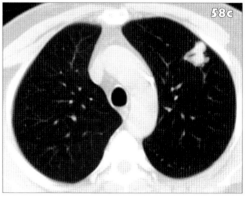

increased when the patient is upright. Patients with hereditary haemorrhagic telangiectasia commonly have nosebleeds and screening is recommended in other family members with similar symptoms. The radiographs may show multiple well-defined nodules with feeding and draining vessels, although some lesions are very small (2–3 mm in diameter) and are best appreciated with CT.

ii. Contrast-enhanced CT or pulmonary angiography is diagnostic, and identifies lesions which may be amenable to embolization (58c). The purpose of treatment is to reduce the right-to-left shunting and therefore the risk of systemic abscess or infarction.

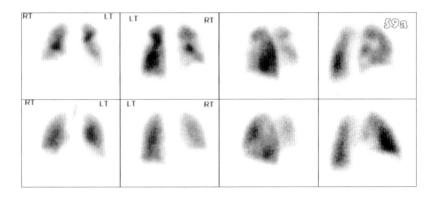

59 A 38-year-old male was recovering from an orthopaedic procedure on his leg. Five days after surgery, he developed sudden onset of pleuritic chest pain. On admission he was hypoxic on air. His chest radiograph was normal. An investigation was performed (59a).
i. What investigation is shown?
ii. What is the diagnosis?

59: Answer

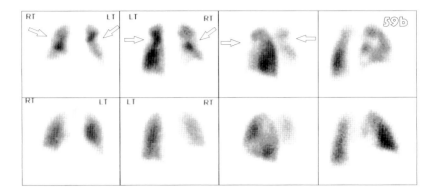

59 i. A ventilation-perfusion (VQ) lung scintigraphy examination is shown. The ventilation study is normal (bottom row of images). The perfusion study (top row of images) shows multiple defects (59b, arrows) which are not seen on the ventilation study (mismatched defects).

ii. The appearances are consistent with a high probability of pulmonary embolus.

The principles of lung scintigraphy involve the imaging of lung perfusion using a radiolabelled tracer which is trapped on first pass in the small capillaries of the lung. Commonly small (10–100µm) particles of macroaggregated human serum albumin (MAA) are used which are labelled with technetium-99m. Lung ventilation is assessed using a radiolabelled inert gas (usually xenon-133 or krypton-81m) or aerosol. The diagnostic abnormality for pulmonary embolus is a defect of pulmonary perfusion in a normally ventilated area of lung, i.e. a mismatched perfusion defect. If pulmonary embolus then leads to infarction, a defect in ventilation is then also seen which is smaller than the perfusion defect. The defects are quantified as subsegmental, segmental, lobar, or even whole lung. When defects do not conform to segmental anatomy, the term nonsegmental is used. A diagnostic algorithm for the interpretation of images has been proposed, classifying the examinations as normal, low probability for PE, intermediate, and high probability. The classification of an abnormal study depends on the number and size of defects and whether they are matched or not.

While a normal study effectively excludes pulmonary embolus and a high probability study is useful for making the diagnosis, the number of indeterminate or intermediate probability studies is high, hence the increased reliance on other techniques such as CT pulmonary angiography.

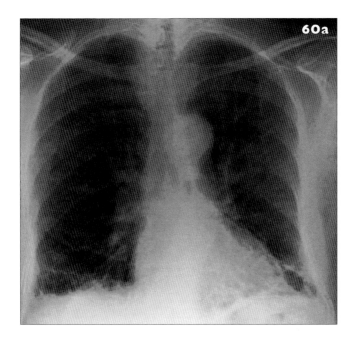

60 A 67-year-old male presented with a history of a recurrent productive cough lasting several years and multiple respiratory tract infections. On examination, he had crepitations at both bases on auscultation. There were no other relevant features on examination and routine blood tests were normal. His chest radiograph is shown (60a).

i. What radiographic features are seen?

ii. What might be expected to be seen on HRCT?

60: Answer

60 i. The chest radiograph shows bilateral lower lobe volume loss, a coarse reticular pattern, and cystic spaces in the lower zones (60a). There is also the impression of 'tram-lining' behind the left heart.

ii. The HRCT shows bilateral varicose bronchiectasis with markedly dilated airways, some of which contain air–fluid levels (60b). The case is an example of the increased specificity of HRCT over chest radiography, in that the differential diagnosis on the radiograph may have

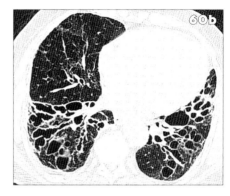

included a basal fibrosing lung disease such as idiopathic pulmonary fibrosis. However, the dilated airways are very well demonstrated on HRCT and are the cause of the cystic spaces on the radiograph.

Bronchiectasis is characterized by local, irreversible dilatation of bronchi, usually accompanied by inflammation. The condition is chronic and patients often present with a persistent cough, recurrent respiratory tract infections, and copious amounts of purulent sputum. Patients may also experience haemoptysis. In the absence of any obvious acquired cause, symptoms can often be traced back to childhood, pre-cipitated by an episode of pneumonia. Macroscopically, bronchiectasis can be classified into cylindrical bronchiectasis where the airway dilatation is mild and the tubular shape of airways is preserved, varicose bronchiectasis where there is dilatation and focal areas of narrowing giving rise to a more irregular, beaded appearance, and cystic (or saccular) bronchiectasis where, as the name suggests, the airway dilatation is almost spherical.

The radiographic appearances of bronchiectasis depend on whether the airway is seen 'en face' or throughout its length. Thickened airway walls are seen as parallel linear opacities (sometimes referred to as 'tram-lines'), whereas ring opacities (sometimes with air–fluid levels) represent airways seen end on. The volume of the lungs varies in relation to the distribution of disease. In widespread forms such as cystic fibrosis, overinflation is often seen, while in localized forms there may be significant volume loss of the affected lobe. The HRCT signs are bronchial dilatation (the diameter of the accompanying pulmonary artery can be used as a reference as it should be the same as the airway), failure of airways to taper peripherally, airways visualized within a centimetre of the pleural surface, and thickening of airway walls. Impacted secretions in and around small peripheral airways may also give rise to 'X'- and 'Y'-shaped small opacities (tree-in-bud pattern). Indirect signs of small airways disease may also be seen (see Question 86).

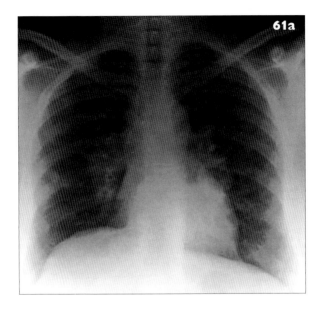

61 A 32-year-old Afro-Caribbean female complained to her family doctor of a rash on her legs. She also had aching joints. She had no respiratory symptoms but a chest radiograph was performed as part of her investigations (61a).
i. What does the radiograph show?
ii. What is the likely diagnosis?
iii. What is the differential diagnosis for the radiographic appearances?

61: Answer

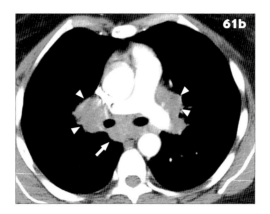

61 i. The chest radiograph shows widening of the mediastinum (in particular, the right paratracheal area) and enlarged lobulated hila bilaterally (61a). The appearances are of mediastinal and bilateral hilar lymphadenopathy. There is also pulmonary nodule in the right mid zone.

ii. The diagnosis is most likely to be sarcoidosis. Erythema nodosum (skin lesions typically involving the shins) often occurs at presentation in patients with sarcoidosis, together with arthralgia and iridocyclitis. The patient had Löfgren's syndrome, a triad consisting of bilateral hilar lymphadenopathy, erythema nodosum, and polyarticular arthritis/arthralgia. Löfgren's syndrome is a characteristic acute form of presentation of sarcoidosis.

iii. The other differential diagnoses to consider in a patient with mediastinal and bilateral hilar lymphadenopathy include tuberculosis, lymphoma, metastases, leukaemia, fungal infection, and a variety of other conditions (e.g. infectious mononucleosis, brucellosis, silicosis, berylliosis, and amyloidosis). Intravenous contrast-enhanced CT shows enlarged subcarinal mediastinal (61b, arrow) and hilar lymph nodes (arrowheads).

Sarcoidosis is a common multisystem disease of unknown aetiology. Histopathologically, sarcoid is characterized by noncaseating epithelioid cell granulomas. Lymphadenopathy is the commonest thoracic manifestation and occurs in the majority at some stage. The lymphadenopathy classically has a symmetric hilar and right paratracheal distribution. The lymph nodes may calcify either in a peripheral (egg-shell) or more subtle diffuse pattern, best appreciated with CT. Most patients (approximately 60%) who present with hilar lymphadenopathy show complete resolution although, in the remainder, parenchymal involvement develops.

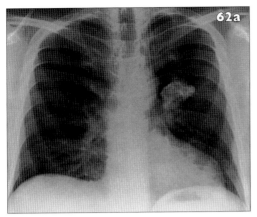
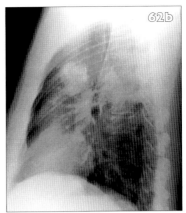

62 A 65-year-old male had a chest radiograph pre-operatively before surgery for an inguinal hernia. He had never smoked. He did not have any respiratory tract symptoms. On examination, his chest was clear. He recalled that a chest radiograph performed 10 years previously had shown an abnormality.

i. What do the PA and lateral chest radiographs (**62a, b**) show?

ii. What investigation should be performed next?

63 A 32-year-old female was being treated with chemotherapy for acute myeloid leukaemia. She was neutropenic and became febrile. No source of infection was found initially, but a small opacity became apparent on her chest radiograph (not shown). An HRCT was performed to characterize the lesion further (**63**).

i. Describe the HRCT findings.

ii. Give a differential diagnosis.

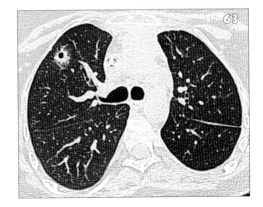

62 i. The PA and lateral chest radiographs show an approximately 4 cm heavily calcified lesion within the anterior segment of the left upper lobe (**62a, b**). It shows the typical 'popcorn-type' calcification of a pulmonary hamartoma. The terms 'hamartochondroma' and 'chondromatous hamartoma' are pathologically more precise. They are regarded as benign lesions and are slow growing and solitary. Hamartomas are usually asymptomatic and the peak age of presentation is in the seventh decade. Pulmonary hamartomas can be up to 10 cm in diameter; however, most are <4 cm in diameter and the larger the lesion, the more likely it is to calcify. The typical 'popcorn-like' cartilage calcification is characteristic but is relatively uncommon, particularly in small lesions. A more common characteristic finding is the presence of focal areas of fat density which can be demonstrated on thin-section CT.
ii. As these lesions are benign, no further investigation or follow-up is necessary.

63 i. The HRCT shows a small peripheral abnormality in the right upper lobe, with a central area of cavitation and an indistinct peripheral margin, a so-called 'halo' of ground-glass opacification (**63**). No other lesions are demonstrated. Note the central venous catheter within the superior vena cava.
ii. The halo sign is due to haemorrhage into the lung around a nodule and the commonest cause is infection, particularly invasive aspergillosis. Other infections to consider would be coccidiomycosis, candidiasis, tuberculosis, cytomegalovirus, and herpes simplex virus. The other noninfectious differential diagnoses for these appearances include Kaposi's sarcoma, Wegener's granulomatosis, and metastatic angiosarcoma. In this case, the appearance was due to invasive aspergillosis.

Invasive aspergillosis is part of a spectrum of pulmonary *Aspergillus fumigatus* infection. It commonly affects immunocompromised hosts and is an angioinvasive process characterized by mycotic vascular invasion, thrombosis, and infarction resulting in cavitation and necrosis. It is the most aggressive form of infection, in comparison with allergic bronchopulmonary aspergillosis (see Question 5), which tends to occur in hyperimmune hosts such as asthmatics, or mycetoma formation in the cavities of individuals with normal immune status. The semi-invasive form is an overlapping condition where there is evidence of angioinvasion in patients with pre-existing cavitary lung disease or emphysema and mild immunocompromise.

The radiographic appearances may be normal in early invasive aspergillosis, and HRCT is more sensitive at detecting the small, ill-defined nodules and areas of cavitation. As the disease develops, widespread areas of consolidation may be seen, which are sometimes rounded and correspond to areas of infarction. On CT, early cavitation may manifest as an air-crescent sign at the upper border of consolidation which then enlarges to form a true cavity. It seems that cavitation is a manifestation of neutrophil recovery, and so paradoxically may be a favourable prognostic sign.

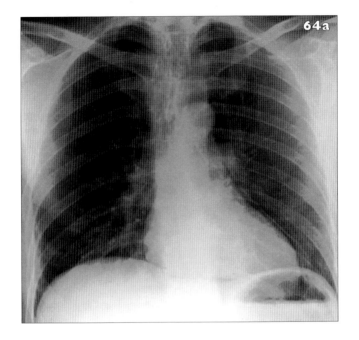

64 An asthmatic had a chest radiograph taken during an acute asthmatic attack (64a).
i. What does it show?
ii. What is the treatment?

64: Answer

64 i. The radiograph shows a pneumomediastinum (air within the mediastinum). The features are relatively subtle but note the air lucency bounded peripherally by a pencil-thin line representing the epicardium (64b, arrows). The sign extends along the undersurface of the heart resulting in the 'continuous diaphragm' sign. Asthmatics may experience a spontaneous alveolar rupture, which results in air in the pleural space, mediastinum, or pericardium.
ii. Depending on the size of the pneumothorax and whether it is under tension, treatment with an intercostal chest drain may be

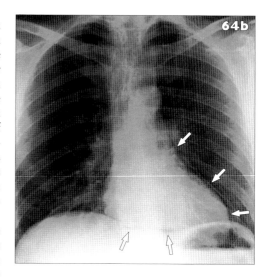

required. A pneumomediastinum or pneumopericardium normally resolves without treatment and tends to be asymptomatic, unless air extends into the soft tissues of the neck, when subcutaneous surgical emphysema may be observed.

In normal individuals, a thin line of apparent lucency may be seen adjacent to the heart border and aortic knuckle. This phenomenon is termed the Mach effect and is a form of optical illusion, where the human eye perceives a much greater lucency at the interface between two structures which differ greatly in attenuation than is actually present. It is possible to differentiate this phenomenon from a pneumomediastinum by the extent and border of the lucency. The Mach effect is adjacent to a normally visualized contour (i.e. will not extend around the inferior border of the heart next to the diaphragm) and the lateral border can be recognized as either a pulmonary vessel or nonexistent. Occasionally, an anterior pneumothorax in a supine patient may cause diagnostic confusion as again air lucency is seen outlining the heart. In these cases, the thin line of the epicardium is not demonstrated and air may be seen to outline the lung over the apex superiorly, or give unusual clarity to the diaphragmatic outline. In difficult cases, a lateral decubitus radiograph may be useful.

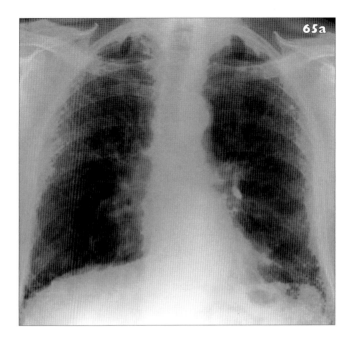

65 A 59-year-old male presented with increasing shortness of breath on exertion and a nonproductive cough over several months. He kept no pets, had worked as a postman since the age of 18 years and was not taking any medication. He had no significant past medical history. On examination, he was clubbed and had late inspiratory crackles on auscultation, particularly at both bases. On lung function tests, he had a restrictive defect with decrease in lung volumes and a decreased gas transfer (DL_{CO}). The radiograph is shown (65a).

Describe the radiological findings.

65: Answer

65 The radiograph shows a slight decrease in lung volumes and a bilateral reticulonodular pattern (65a). There is also the impression of bilateral small cyst-like translucencies, a few millimetres in diameter, so-called 'honeycomb lung'. The features are more clearly demonstrated on HRCT where there is a basal, subpleural predominance of cysts or honeycombing (65b–d). A more subtle subpleural reticular pattern is seen in the upper zones. There is distortion of the architecture of the lung and the airways adjacent to the honeycomb pattern are dilated by the fibrosis, a finding known as 'traction bronchiectasis' (65d, arrow).

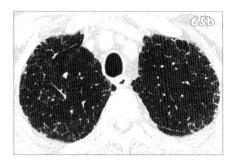

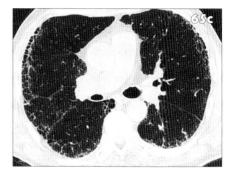

The clinical and radiological features are those of idiopathic pulmonary fibrosis (IPF). By definition, there is no antecedent cause and the condition usually occurs in adults in the fifth or sixth decade. IPF is a relatively uncommon condition, occurring in 3–5 patients per 100,000 population. The prognosis is poor, with a mean survival of 4.5 years after presentation. The commonest histopathological subtype is usual interstitial pneumonitis (UIP), which is characterized by a patchy distribution of established fibrosis, fibroblastic foci, and normal lung. The radiological features of UIP are characterized by basal reticulonodular shadowing on the radiograph and a predominantly subpleural and basal reticular pattern and honeycombing on HRCT.

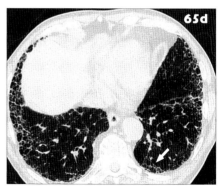

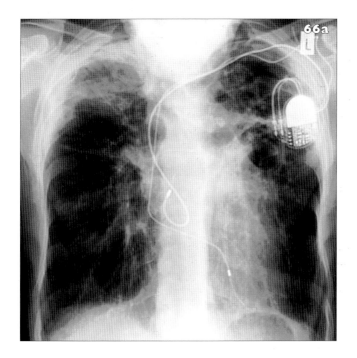

66 A 68-year-old male presented with haemoptysis. He had been a heavy smoker in the past. He had a history of pulmonary tuberculosis (TB) and had had a permanent pacemaker inserted for symptomatic episodes of complete heart block. On examination, he was well, not clubbed or cyanosed, and had some crackles bilaterally on auscultation of the upper and mid zones.
i. What does the chest radiograph show (66a)?
ii. What is the likely cause of the haemoptysis?

66: Answer

66 i. The chest radiograph shows bilateral upper lobe volume loss and fibrocavitary disease due to his previous pulmonary TB. There is a dual chamber permanent cardiac pacemaker *in situ*. At the right apex, there is increased soft tissue density within one of the cavities, with an air crescent sign superiorly (**66b**, arrows). Note the marked pleural thickening laterally. The HRCT shows an intracavitary fungus ball, again with a rim of surrounding air (**66c**, arrows).

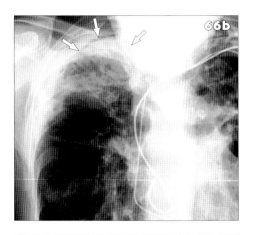

ii. The findings are typical of a mycetoma or aspergilloma. The formation of a mycetoma is due to saprophytic colonization of a pre-existing chronic cavity with *Aspergillus fumigatus*. The initial cavity is usually due to TB or sarcoidosis. Other causes include previous *Pneumocystis carinii* infection, ankylosing spondylitis, and histoplasmosis. There are even reports of mycetoma formation in a cavity due to a neoplastic process. The

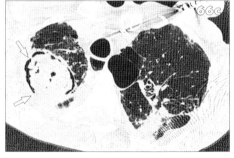

patient may be asymptomatic, but may also present with haemoptysis as in the current case. Microscopic examination reveals hyphae which do not invade adjacent pulmonary parenchyma unless there is host immunocompromise. The exact cause of bleeding in these cases is not known, although various theories have been postulated including friction between the fungus ball and the inflamed wall of the cavity.

The radiographic appearances reflect the fact that most of the cavities that are colonized occur in the upper lobes. The air crescent sign is typical but not absolutely pathognomonic and the fungus ball may be seen to be mobile on radiography (including tomography) or CT. Adjacent pleural thickening is very common and may be an early sign of aspergilloma formation. The CT appearances are often very helpful in suggesting the diagnosis because of the lack of superimposed parenchyma in patients with chronic lung disease. The fungus ball is seen to consist of a sponge-like mass with internal air densities and surrounding air lucency between the fungus ball and the wall of the cavity. In cases with recurrent haemoptysis, radiologically-guided injection of antifungals or wax may be useful in controlling symptoms.

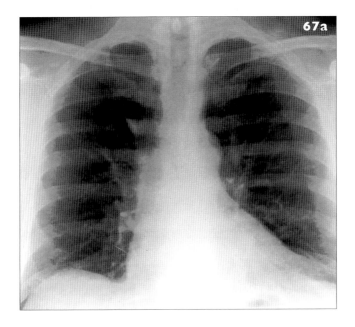

67 A 50-year-old male presented with a dry cough for 5 months which commenced after a coryzal illness. He smoked 20 cigarettes per day but had recently cut down. He appeared clinically well and examination of the respiratory system was normal. Blood tests, including a full blood count and urea and electrolytes, were normal. He had normal respiratory function at spirometry.

What normal variant is demonstrated on the radiograph (67a)?

67 The PA chest radiograph shows a fine linear opacity laterally, with a thicker density inferiorly adjacent to the right superior mediastinum (**67a**). The azygos arch is not seen in its usual site immediately superior to the right main bronchus, but a density is seen more superiorly at the base of the fine linear opacity. The normal variant shown is an azygos lobe and fissure.

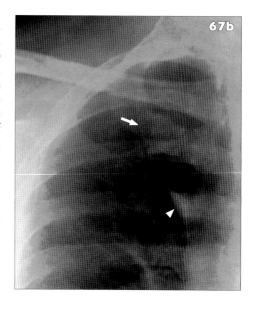

An azygos lobe occurs in 0.4–1% of the population, based on both clinical and post-mortem studies. A familial occurrence has been described and there is evidence that it is commoner in males. On the frontal chest radiograph, a hairline curvilinear opacity is seen which extends across the right upper zone obliquely and is concave to the mediastinum (**67b**, arrow). Where it originates peripherally, a triangular small soft tissue opacity may be seen (trigonum parietale) (**67b**, arrowhead). The teardrop-shaped opacity of the azygos vein is usually seen inferiorly within the fissure, displaced from the normal position in the angle between the right main bronchus and trachea. It results from failure of migration of the azygos vein from the chest wall to the normal position in the tracheobronchial angle. The azygos fissure supports the azygos vein in a sling and consists of four layers of pleura (two parietal and two visceral), unlike other fissures which consist of two layers of visceral pleura. The term azygos lobe is a misnomer as this portion of lung is supplied by branches of the apical or posterior segmental bronchus of the upper lobe.

The azygos lobe is not unduly susceptible to disease but may occupy less volume than a normally configured right upper lobe. Overlap of supra-aortic vessels may also cause the azygos lobe to appear rather opaque, which may simulate a mediastinal mass or even right upper lobe collapse.

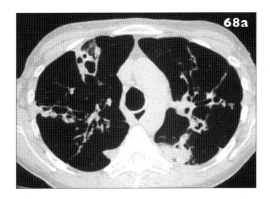

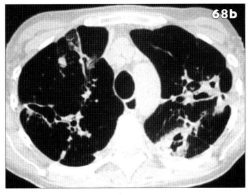

68 A 60-year-old female developed a cough productive of yellow sputum with intermittent haemoptyses over the next few years. This was associated with a gradual decline in exercise tolerance. She was a life-long nonsmoker and had mild rheumatoid arthritis. On examination, coarse crepitations were audible in both lungs, most prominently at the bases. Multiple sputum smears and cultures were persistently positive for acid-fast bacilli, despite prolonged courses (up to 4 years) of antimicrobial therapy. Ethambutol was intermittently removed from the drug regime due to problems with optic nerve toxicity. Over a 10-year period her FEV_1 declined from 1.6 l to 1.3 l and her FVC from 2.9 l to 1.9 l. Her gas transfer (K_{CO}) remained fairly static at around 50–60% of that predicted.
i. What does the HRCT show (**68a, b**)?
ii. What diagnosis should be suggested?

68: Answer

68 i. The HRCT images demonstrate bronchiectasis, areas of consolidation with cavitation, and the occasional nodular opacity (**68a, b**).

ii. Infection with an atypical or nontuberculous mycobacterium should be considered. The patient was subsequently found to be infected with *Mycobacterium avium intracellulare* (MAI), the commonest of the nontuberculous mycobacteria (NTM) species. Other well-recognized species causing pulmonary disease include *M. kansasii* and *M. xenopi*, with several others such as *M. malmoense*, *M. chelonae*, and *M. fortuitum* playing a less well-understood role. MAI is a common opportunistic pathogen in AIDS patients. Most NTM organisms have been isolated from soil and water and are not thought to be transmitted from person to person.

Radiological patterns of disease are disparate. NTM are low-grade pathogens and often infect patients with existing lung disease such as emphysema, chronic obstructive airways disease, and previous *M. tuberculosis* infection. However, three 'characteristic' patterns can be distinguished:

- MAI infection: small nodules and bronchiectasis are the hallmark of infection by this organism, with cavitation in approximately 30%. It is now believed that bronchiectasis is the consequence of chronic MAI infection over the years rather than the organism colonizing already affected airways.
- *M. kansasii* and *M. xenopi* infection: there is less consensus on the radiographic patterns caused by these organisms. However, cavities are present in 61–96% and are usually apical or subapical in location (and thus resemble conventional active TB). Nodules, fibrosis, and infiltrates are also seen in a few patients.
- Immunocompromised patients (including AIDS): there is often prominent mediastinal and hilar lymphadenopathy but no parenchymal disease. Non-AIDS patients may demonstrate miliary nodules and cavitation. Importantly, adenopathy (and pleural effusions) are rare in immunocompetent patients, and their presence should raise the possibility of other disease such as *M. tuberculosis*.

Diagnostic criteria for invasive disease, rather than colonization by these organisms, are debated. The American Thoracic Society guidelines are widely accepted and require moderate to heavy growth of the organism from repeated sputum specimens in the context of appropriate clinical and radiological findings. Bronchoalveolar lavage and/or transbronchial biopsy specimens further increase the yield. Treatment is difficult. *M. kansasii* and *M. xenopi* are relatively easy to treat with a combination of isoniazid, rifampicin (rifampin), and ethambutol. MAI, however, is difficult to eradicate, with a high percentage of cases relapsing on cessation of treatment.

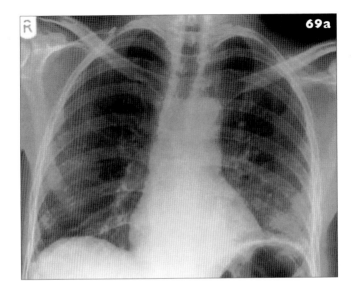

69 A 32-year-old male presented with sudden onset of mild chest pain, palpitations, dizziness, and sweating, followed by loss of consciousness and a witnessed seizure. He had injured his right ankle 2 weeks previously and had noticed a recent pain in his right calf. On examination, he was sweaty, cool, and poorly perfused. He was tachycardic with a pulse of 140, normotensive, and tachypnoeic with a respiratory rate of 38. His JVP was elevated. His left base was dull to percussion with decreased air entry. His arterial blood gases (on 15 l/min O_2) were: pH: 7.50; pCO_2: 22.5 mmHg (3.0 kPa); pO_2: 75.7 mmHg (10.1 kPa); HCO_3^-: 18 mmol/l; oxygen saturation: 97%. His ECG showed sinus tachycardia.
i. What does the chest radiograph show (69a)?
ii. What radiological investigation should be performed next?

69: Answer

69 i. The PA chest radiograph shows subtle patchy consolidation in the left lower zone, with some volume loss as denoted by the high left hemidiaphragm (**69a**).

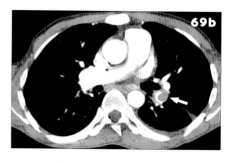

ii. The next imaging investigation of choice would be either a CT pulmonary angiogram or ventilation-perfusion scintigraphy. The CT pulmonary angiogram shows large filling defects within the left lower lobe pulmonary artery and

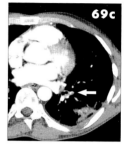

the left lower lobe segmental branches (**69b, c,** arrows). There is patchy parenchymal opacification in the left lower lobe which represents pulmonary haemorrhage, with or without infarction. There is a small left pleural effusion.

The radiographic signs of pulmonary embolism are nonspecific and the chest radiograph is insensitive in the detection of acute pulmonary embolus. If there is no infarction or haemorrhage present, there may be oligaemia or vessel 'cut-off' in the lung distal to the embolus (Westermark's sign), with increase in the diameter of the pulmonary artery proximal to the thrombus. There may also be volume loss, with elevation of the diaphragm. Adjacent linear areas of atelectasis can also be a feature. If pulmonary infarction is present, radiographic consolidation may be seen. A 'Hampton's hump' refers to a peripheral wedge-shaped area of opacification which contacts the pleural surface at its base. Cavitation within the infarct is rare, and although it may occur in noninfected infarcts, it is more common with secondary infection or septic emboli.

The major role of the chest radiograph is to exclude diagnoses which may mimic the clinical picture of pulmonary embolism (such as pneumothorax, pneumonia, and dissecting aortic aneurysm) and to provide a baseline to assist in the interpretation of a subsequent ventilation-perfusion (VQ) scan. The PIOPED study showed that a high probability scan (a perfusion scan showing multiple segmental defects with a normal ventilation scan, so-called mismatched perfusion defects) or a normal scan are both very accurate at diagnosing or excluding pulmonary embolism, respectively. Unfortunately, the majority of patients fall outside this group and are classified as indeterminate. In this large group of patients, pulmonary angiography (the traditional 'gold standard') was formerly advocated to establish the diagnosis. However, CT pulmonary angiography (CTPA) has largely supplanted traditional pulmonary angiography and is also able to image thrombus directly within the vessel lumen. Thrombus is seen as either a partial filling defect or complete occlusion of the vessel (which may be expanded by clot).

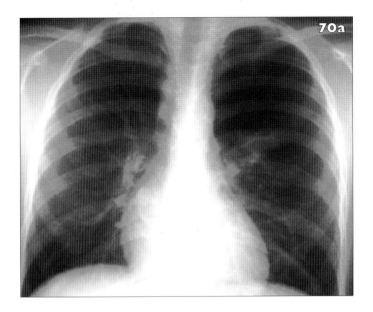

70 A 9-year-old male presented with recurrent left-sided pneumonia requiring antibiotic treatment. Past medical history included chickenpox infection and episodes of tonsillitis. On examination, he was well, not clubbed or cyanosed. He had reduced breath sounds anteriorly in the left upper zone but otherwise examination was unremarkable. Spirometry was normal.

What abnormalities are demonstrated on the chest radiograph (70a)?

70: Answer

70 The chest radiograph demonstrates hyperlucency of the left upper zone. There is a subtle 3.5 cm diameter lobulated opacity in the left upper zone which is well defined, thin-walled superiorly, and contains an air–fluid level (70b, arrow). The CT scan demonstrates a hyperlucent left upper lobe (70c). There are a reduced number of normal bronchovascular structures within this part of the lung and several bronchi (arrow) were slightly dilated. The opacity demonstrated on the chest radiograph is central and adjacent to the superior pole of the left hilum. The apicoposterior segmental bronchus is not seen separately and again an air–fluid level is demonstrated on CT. Appearances are those of congenital bronchial atresia. The patient subsequently underwent a left upper lobectomy and histopathological examination was confirmatory.

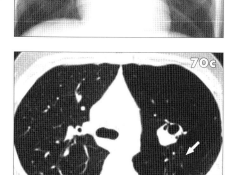

Bronchial atresia is a rare congenital anomaly. Patients may present with recurrent chest infections as in this case, but at least 50% are asymptomatic and the abnormality is discovered as an incidental finding. The commonest lobe to be affected is the left upper lobe (64%), followed by the left lower lobe (14%), and the right middle and lower lobes (8%). Involvement of more than one lung segment is extremely rare. The anomaly is due to focal obliteration of a proximal segmental or subsegmental bronchus, with normal development of distal structures. A bronchocele results from accumulation of mucus within distal bronchi. The lung distal to the atretic bronchus is underventilated: ventilation occurs by collateral air drift and the surrounding lung is hyperlucent; air trapping may be confirmed on expiratory radiographs or CT. The diagnosis can often be made on the plain radiograph: typically the bronchocele is a rounded, branching opacity adjacent to the hilum surrounded by hyperlucent lung. As demonstrated in this case, an air–fluid level sometimes occurs, but this is rare. CT demonstrates the features more elegantly than chest radiography and allows more accurate delineation of lobar anatomy. On MRI, a bronchocele characteristically returns high signal on both T1- and T2-weighted images, although the disadvantage of the technique is its inability to demonstrate the surrounding hyperlucent lung.

The differential diagnosis includes congenital cystic adenomatoid malformation, or a bronchogenic cyst, but surrounding pulmonary hyperlucency is not an expected feature.

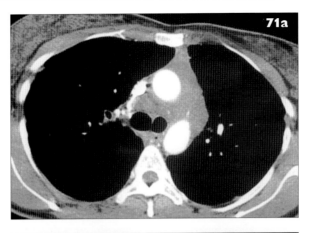

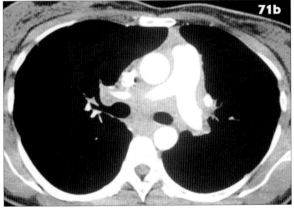

71 A 28-year-old female presented with a 3-month history of progressive dyspnoea. She had had a diagnosis of pulmonary sarcoidosis made 5 years previously and was a lifelong nonsmoker. On examination she was slightly tachypnoeic, but no other abnormality was demonstrated. Routine blood tests and lung function tests were normal. An intravenous contrast-enhanced CT is shown (71a, b).
i. What abnormality is seen?
ii. List the possible causes.

71: Answer

71 i. The CT images show increased soft tissue attenuation of the mediastinal fat (71a, b). The mediastinal fat should have the same density as subcutaneous fat, but it is grossly abnormal in this case due to extensive infiltration of the mediastinum by abnormal soft tissue which encases the great vessels and major airways. It is not possible to identify discrete lymph nodes.

ii. The CT appearances are typical of fibrosing mediastinitis although neoplastic infiltration is another possible cause. Fibrosing mediastinitis is a rare condition, characterized by chronic inflammation and fibrosis of mediastinal soft tissues. The most common causes are histoplasmosis, tuberculosis, and sarcoidosis (the cause in this case). The precise pathogenesis of the fibrotic reaction is unclear. The possibilities include spillage of necrotic material from infected nodes inciting an inflammatory reaction with secondary fibrosis, or an idiosyncratic hypersensitivity reaction to the presence of organisms or associated necrotic material. Nevertheless, a considerable number of cases are idiopathic. An autoimmune aetiology has been proposed for this latter group, some of whom have similar fibrotic processes in other anatomic sites, such as the retroperitoneum (retroperitoneal fibrosis), thyroid (Riedel's struma), orbit (orbital pseudotumour), and the caecum (ligneous perityphlitis).

Fibrosing mediastinitis is seen on CT as replacement of the mediastinal fat by infiltrating soft tissue in which discrete enlarged lymph nodes cannot be identified. Compression and/or encasement of the trachea, main bronchi, and mediastinal vessels is common. Obstruction of the superior vena cava (SVC) is probably the most common cause of clinical symptoms (SVC syndrome), although symptoms often improve with the development of collaterals. Narrowing of the trachea and main bronchi is common and, in association with narrowing and/or obstruction of the central pulmonary arteries and veins, frequently results in pulmonary parenchymal infiltrates (atelectasis/collapse, consolidation, infarction), and pleural effusions. Two distinctly different patterns of disease are recognized:

- Localized pattern of fibrosis which frequently contains calcification. This is the most common pattern. In the USA, this is usually due to histoplasmosis and little benefit is derived from steroid therapy.
- Less common pattern of a diffuse homogeneous soft-tissue process, infiltrating the mediastinum but with no calcification (as in this case). These cases are more commonly idiopathic and sometimes improve with steroid treatment.

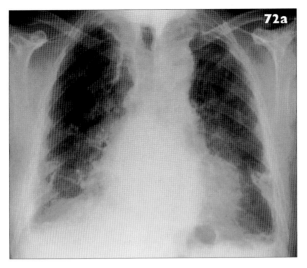

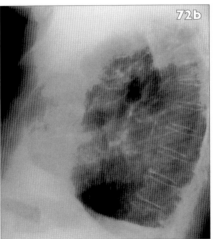

72 An 85-year-old male presented with dysphagia and weight loss. He had been fit and well previously and was a retired electrician. He was an ex-smoker and drank alcohol in moderation. On examination of his respiratory system, no abnormality was found. He had a mild normochromic normocytic anaemia on full blood count. His frontal and lateral chest radiographs are shown (**72a, b**).

What radiographic abnormalities are present?

72: Answer

72 The frontal radiograph shows bilateral calcified pleural thickening, consistent with his previous asbestos exposure (72a). In addition, there is a subtle increase in density of the central inferior mediastinum behind the heart. On the lateral view, there is a posterior mediastinal mass (72c, arrows). The large mass is best appreciated on CT (72d) where there is anterior displacement of the heart and, although the mass contacts the margin of the descending thoracic aorta, is seen not to originate from this structure. The oesophagus is not seen separately but appears to be markedly deviated to the left as denoted by a tiny fleck of gas at the margin of the mass. The mass is seen to be of homogeneous soft-tissue attenuation, with no contrast enhancement. The lesion was biopsied and found to be a large cell undifferentiated carcinoma, probably of lung origin.

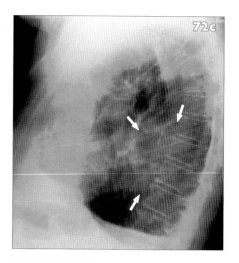

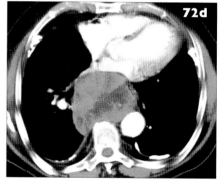

The differential diagnosis of a posterior mediastinal mass in adults is discussed in Question 77. This case demonstrates how a very large mass behind the heart may be easily missed on a PA radiograph. An azygo-oesophageal line is normally seen behind the heart on a PA radiograph and represents the interface between aerated lung within the right lower lobe, and the right wall of the oesophagus and azygos vein. Convexity or absence of the line is suspicious of a subcarinal mass.

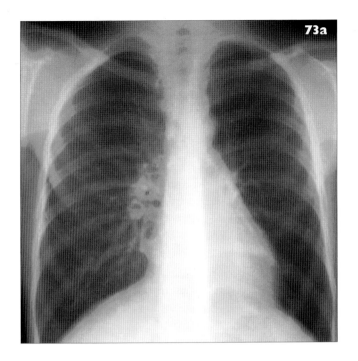

73 A 13-year-old male was investigated for recurrent respiratory infections. He had had several episodes of repeated lower respiratory tract infections from the age of 15 months and since that time had been troubled by a productive cough and wheezing. Cystic fibrosis, ciliary dyskinesia, and an immunodeficiency had been excluded. Relevant immunizations were up to date. He had an elder sister who was well, and the family did not keep any pets. On examination, he was well. There was no clubbing or cyanosis; breath sounds were reduced on the left side with a few crackles at the left base and also wheezes on the right. His pulmonary function tests indicated an obstructive lung disease (% of predicted values): FVC: 76%; FEV$_1$: 46 %; FEV$_1$/FVC: -35%.

What does the chest radiograph show (73a)?

73: Answer

73 The chest radiograph demonstrates a hyperlucent, slightly small left lung with reduced vascular markings compared to the right lung (73a). The left pulmonary artery is also smaller than the right. There is the suggestion of bronchial wall thickening in the left lower lobe. A bronchogram was performed some time previously, and demonstrated a decreased number of bronchial divisions in the left lung, with peripheral 'pruning' of the bronchial tree consistent with obliterative bronchiolitis (73b). An HRCT study was obtained. The images show the entire left lung is of decreased attenuation by comparison with the right (73c, d). The vessels within the areas of decreased attenuation are of reduced calibre and the left pulmonary arterial branches are markedly reduced in size. The airways within the left lower lobe are slightly dilated and thick-walled (73d, arrows). The imaging features are those of Macleod's (Swyer-James') syndrome.

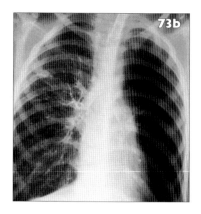

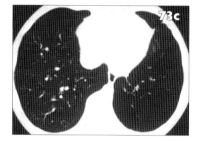

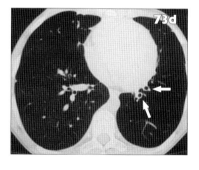

Macleod's (Swyer–James') syndrome is a variant of post-infectious, constrictive obliterative bronchiolitis. By definition, the small airways disease, as demonstrated by the chest radiograph, is concentrated in one lung giving rise to the cardinal sign of unilateral hyper-transradiancy. It results from an acute bronchiolitis (usually viral) in infancy or childhood, resulting in damage to the terminal and respiratory bronchioles and prevention of the normal development of distal alveolar buds. The reduction of pulmonary circulation is thought to be secondary to alveolar damage. The condition is usually asymptomatic in adulthood, but cough, repeated pulmonary infections, and haemoptysis have been described. The usual radiographic features are of a unilateral hyperlucent lobe or lung of reduced volume and reduced peripheral and central pulmonary vasculature. However, depending on the timing of the insult, the lung volume and radiographic density may be normal. Air-trapping is demonstrated on expiratory radiographs.

HRCT shows these features more elegantly than chest radiography and is a more sensitive method of detecting bronchiectasis than the chest radiograph.

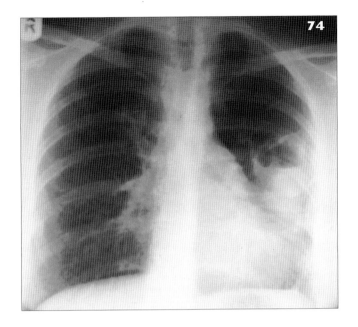

74 A 30-year-old female presented with stridor, cough and haemoptysis, night sweats, and arthralgia. Her initial presentation was at the age of 22 years with recurrent ear infections, epistaxis, malaise, and weight loss. She was a lifelong nonsmoker. On examination, she had inspiratory stridor. The lungs were clear on auscultation. She had significant hearing loss bilaterally. Blood tests showed a raised CRP and ESR. Urea and creatinine were normal.

i. What does the radiograph show (74)?
ii. What is the radiological differential diagnosis?
iii. What pathological features might be expected on nasal biopsy?

74: Answer

74 i. The PA chest radiograph shows a large lesion in the left mid zone with an air–fluid level consistent with a cavity (74).

ii. The differential diagnosis on the basis of the imaging alone includes abscess, tuberculosis, cavitating carcinoma, pulmonary infarct, necrotic rheumatoid nodule, cavitating metastasis, and Wegener's granulomatosis. The cANCA was positive in this case.

iii. Nasal biopsy (at initial presentation) showed necrotizing granulomas in the walls of small blood vessels with a lymphocytic infiltrate, consistent with Wegener's granulomatosis.

Wegener's granulomatosis is a necrotizing granulomatous vasculitis which involves the upper and lower respiratory tracts and, in the classic form, there is a focal necrotizing glomerulonephritis. Other organs are involved to a variable extent by a small vessel granulomatous vasculitis. Approximately one-fifth of patients do not have renal or other extrapulmonary involvement. This uncommon disease can occur at any age but the mean age at presentation is 40 years with a male to female ratio of 3:2. ANCA are strongly positive in the small vessel vasculitides and 85% of patients with untreated Wegener's granulomatosis have cANCA positivity. The clinical presentation is variable and often consists of nonspecific constitutional symptoms. However, respiratory tract symptoms and signs predominate.

The classic radiographic finding is of multiple pulmonary nodules of variable size (range 3–70 mm), frequently cavitating. More diffuse pulmonary involvement, ranging from bilateral ground-glass opacification to areas of dense consolidation, are also common. Diffuse bilateral consolidation due to widespread pulmonary haemorrhage and pleural effusions may occur. CT allows further characterization of nodules shown on radiography, and frequently reveals further radiographically occult lesions. The nodules have a random distribution throughout the lungs but are reported to be usually in close proximity to pulmonary vessels. Bronchiectasis and bronchial wall thickening have also been reported as relatively frequent findings. Tracheal narrowing may occur resulting in a localized stenosis, often subglottic in location.

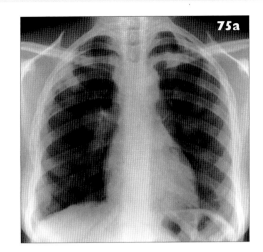

75 A 29-year-old Afro-Caribbean female presented to her family doctor feeling nonspecifically unwell with a nonproductive cough and arthralgia. Her symptoms had been present for several weeks. There were no abnormalities on physical examination and she was apyrexial. Full blood count and urea and electrolytes were normal.

A chest radiograph was performed (75a).

i. What are the findings?

ii. What are the differential diagnoses?

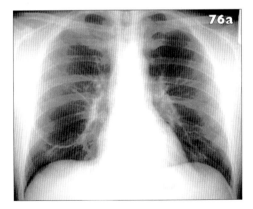

76 A 31-year-old male presented with recurrent chest infections requiring antibiotic treatment since childhood. After two episodes of pneumonia in 6 months, he was referred for further investigation by his family doctor. On examination, he was well and had no symptoms at the time of the chest radiograph or CT scan (76a, b).

i. What are the findings?

ii. What is a possible diagnosis?

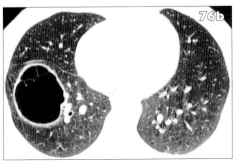

75, 76: Answers

75 i. The chest radiograph shows large, bilateral pulmonary nodules of varying size (75a). An upper- and mid-zone distribution is demonstrated. There is no obvious cavitation and no pleural effusion. The nodules are slightly ill-defined. There is the impression of bilateral and mediastinal lymphadenopathy.

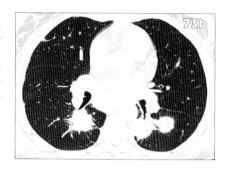

ii. The differential diagnoses include sarcoidosis, metastases, infection, Wegener's granulomatosis, and rheumatoid nodules.

The diagnosis of pulmonary sarcoidosis was made in this case by transbronchial biopsy.

Large nodules are an uncommon but well-recognized manifestation of pulmonary sarcoidosis, occurring in approximately 2–3% of cases. The nodules range from 5 mm to 5 cm in diameter, and are usually multiple. They may be slightly ill-defined or irregular as in this case, and may also show air bronchograms or, very rarely, cavitation. Most coexist with mediastinal and hilar lymphadenopathy. The nodules may completely or partially regress or persist over long periods of time.

The HRCT shows the rather irregular stellate margins of the nodules and the close relationship with adjacent airways (75b).

76 i. The chest radiograph shows a well-defined thin-walled cystic lesion in the right mid zone (76a). The CT confirms the findings and the lesion is seen within the right lower lobe (76b).

ii. A post-infective pneumatocele would be the differential diagnosis. A right lower lobectomy was performed and a diagnosis of congenital cystic adenomatoid malformation was made histopathologically.

Congenital cystic adenomatoid malformation (CCAM) is a rare condition which usually presents in neonates and may be life-threatening. Occasionally, CCAM presents in adults (as in this case). The developmental abnormality occurs *in utero* and consists of a hamartomatous mass of fibrous tissue and smooth muscle, containing cystic spaces lined by columnar or cuboidal respiratory epithelium. There are three basic types: Type 1 consists of one or more cysts >2 cm in diameter; Type 2 contains cysts <2 cm in diameter; and Type 3 is macroscopically solid. Type 1 CCAM has the best prognosis. The process usually involves one lung lobe and may be expansile, resulting in neonatal respiratory distress.

Normally, the chest radiograph shows a mass involving a hemithorax with evidence of pressure effects on surrounding structures. There may be multiple air–fluid levels within the cysts, although a single cyst may be predominant. The CT often shows multiple cystic areas. Other causes of focal cystic areas in the lung are pneumatoceles and hydatid disease, but pneumatoceles do not generally form clusters and hydatid cysts tend to be fluid-filled.

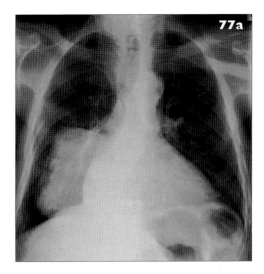

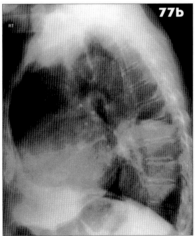

77 An 82-year-old male had a routine chest radiograph prior to an inguinal hernia repair operation. He had been a smoker in the past and had a history of hypertension. On examination, he was well with a slightly raised blood pressure (175/110 mmHg; 23.3/14.7 kPa). A short systolic murmur was noted on auscultation of his precordium but otherwise examination was unremarkable. His frontal and lateral chest radiographs are shown (77a, b).

i. What are the findings?

ii. What radiological investigation should be performed next?

77: Answer

77 i. The frontal radiograph shows a large, well-defined mass in the right hemithorax which is not obscuring the right heart border or the right hemidiaphragm (77a). There is cardiomegaly. The lateral radiograph shows the mass to be within the posterior mediastinum (77b). The differential diagnosis for posterior mediastinal masses includes a dilated oesophagus or hiatus hernia (although no fluid level is demonstrated), oesophageal duplication cyst, and unfolding, aneursym or rupture of the descending thoracic aorta. Paravertebral posterior mediastinal masses tend to be projected over the spine and include bony metastases, extramedullary haemopoiesis, abscess, and neurogenic tumours in adults.

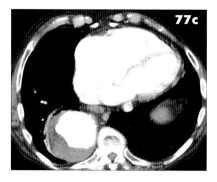

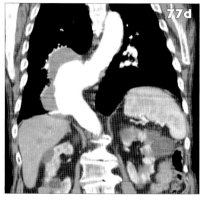

ii. A CT would be the next investigation of choice. CT shows the descending thoracic aorta projected to the right of the thoracic spine (normally on the left) consistent with ectasia or unfolding (77c). In addition, the thoracic aorta is dilated and the lumen consists of both flowing blood (showing as white on the intravenous contrast-enhanced CT) and soft tissue attenuation, which represents mural thrombus. The coronal reformatted image shows the craniocaudal extent of the aneurysm (77d).

For many years, aortography, where a catheter is placed directly into an artery, was the imaging investigation of choice. More recently, CT, MRI, and ultrasound (including transoesophageal ultrasound) are used as accurate noninvasive techniques able to assess the thoracic aorta. Most patients are hypertensive and chest pain and compression effects are the commonest presenting features, although a significant proportion (as in the current case) are discovered incidentally. A hoarse voice from compression of the recurrent laryngeal nerve, collapse of the left lower lobe from compression of the left lower lobe or left main bronchus, or dysphagia from oesophageal compression are all described. The majority of degenerative aneurysms show some intraluminal thrombus which forms a crescent shape against the wall of the aorta. The thrombus may also be calcified and peripheral curvilinear calcification can be a useful sign on radiography to distinguish the abnormality as being vascular in origin.

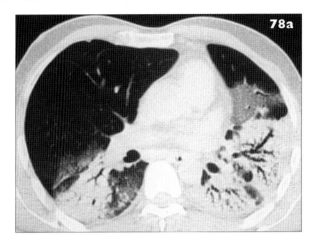

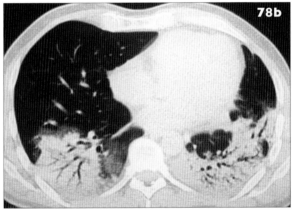

78 A 55-year-old male presented with fatigue, joint pains, and an influenza-like illness. He had several chest radiographs (not shown) which showed bilateral shadowing that persisted over several weeks, despite multiple courses of anti-biotics. On examination, he was not clubbed but had bilateral crepitations on auscultation. His routine blood tests were normal, apart from a raised ESR and CRP. His HRCT is shown (78a, b).

i. Describe the findings.
ii. What is the likely diagnosis?

78: Answer

78 i. The HRCT shows bilateral basal areas of dense consolidation with prominent air bronchograms (78a, b). There is some surrounding ground-glass opacification. The airways appear slightly dilated within the areas of consolidation, suggestive of an element of fibrosis.

ii. Although infection is a possibility, the fact that the patient had persisting abnormality on the chest radiograph for several months makes this unlikely. The prime diagnosis is an organizing pneumonia or bronchioloalveolar cell carcinoma; other possibilities include an eosinophilic pneumonia or lymphoma. The patient subsequently underwent an open lung biopsy and the histopathological diagnosis of an organizing pneumonia was made.

Organizing pneumonia is regarded as a reparative response to an insult and may be seen in a variety of conditions. The entity used to be synonymous with bronchiolitis obliterans organizing pneumonia (BOOP), but the term organizing pneumonia is now favoured to avoid confusion with the completely separate entity of obliterative bronchiolitis. The histopathological characteristics of organizing pneumonia are patchy cellular fibrosis that occludes alveoli, alveolar ducts, and sometimes terminal bronchioles. The cellular infiltrate within the matrix consists of lymphocytes, plasma cells, macrophages, and neutrophils which may conglomerate into an elongated structure (the characteristic Masson body). An organizing pneumonia may either be cryptogenic, a nonspecific finding bordering unrelated pathology (e.g. neoplasms, abscesses), or a minor component of other diseases (e.g. extrinsic allergic alveolitis).

Cryptogenic organizing pneumonia (COP) is a rare condition which often presents as an influenza-like illness and, because of the accompanying radiographic consolidation, is often initially misdiagnosed as an infective pneumonia. The radiographic abnormality may however, persist, migrate, or even wax and wane without treatment. Some studies have suggested that there is a basal or peripheral predominance, although CT may also show a bronchovascular distribution of consolidation. On CT there may also be small nodules or ground-glass opacities. There is spontaneous resolution in some cases, but most require treatment with corticosteroids.

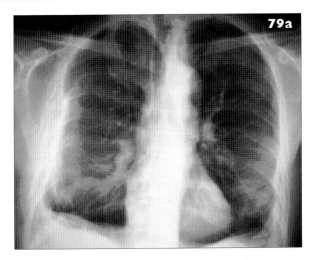

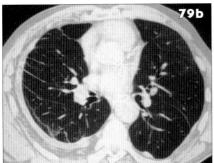
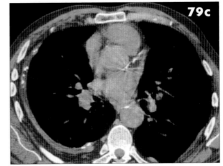

79 A 62-year-old male presented with decreasing exercise tolerance and shortness of breath. He had no other respiratory symptoms. He had worked in shipyards, maintaining boilers for 15 years when he had been heavily exposed to asbestos. Seventeen years had elapsed since his last exposure. He was not clubbed, cyanosed, or breathless at rest. Auscultation of his chest revealed no added sounds although the breath sounds were quiet. Full blood count and biochemistry were normal. His lung function tests showed a restrictive defect with a total lung capacity (TLC) 65% of predicted and a raised adjusted gas transfer coefficient (K_{CO}) of 115% of predicted. The RV/TLC ratio was slightly raised (110% of predicted).

i. What do the chest radiograph (79a) and HRCT (79b, c) show?
ii. What is the likely cause?

79: Answer

79 i. The chest radiograph shows bilateral pleural thickening which blunts the costophrenic angles and extends up the lateral chest wall internal to the ribs (79a). The pleural thickening is calcified on the right, with a rather well-circumscribed, straight border medially. Parenchymal bands can be seen contacting both pleural surfaces. The HRCT shows predominantly right-sided, smooth, diffuse pleural thickening which was more extensive posterobasally where bilateral pleural thickening was also seen (lower images not shown) (79b, c). There is volume loss of the right hemithorax and increased extrapleural fat. There are parenchymal bands contacting the pleural surface, so-called 'crow's feet'. There is also thickening of both oblique fissures. There is some parenchymal distortion related to the pleural disease, but no parenchymal interstitial fibrosis.

ii. The appearances are typical of diffuse pleural thickening secondary to asbestos exposure. The differential diagnosis of symmetrical, bilateral, uniform pleural thickening is limited but includes drug-related disease (particularly amiodarone) and the rare condition of cryptogenic fibrosing pleuritis.

Diffuse pleural thickening results from thickening and fibrosis of the visceral pleura, with fusion to the parietal pleura, often over a wide area. Many studies have confirmed that diffuse pleural thickening is preceded by a benign asbestos pleural effusion. The exposure–response relationship for diffuse pleural thickening is considered to be similar to that of pleural plaques in that it is related to time since first exposure. The latent period is approximately 15 years and the progression of diffuse pleural thickening is slow.

Diffuse pleural thickening has been radiographically defined as a smooth non-interrupted pleural density extending over at least one-quarter of the chest wall, with or without costophrenic angle obliteration. The equivalent CT definition is a continuous sheet of pleural thickening >5 cm wide, >8 cm in craniocaudal extent, and >3 mm in thickness. Diffuse pleural thickening which is <3 mm thick or less extensive may still be functionally significant, however, and a less rigorous definition is probably more appropriate.

Differentiation from pleural plaques can sometimes be difficult. However, plaques generally spare the costophrenic angles and apices. Diffuse pleural thickening is ill-defined and irregular from all angles whereas plaques are often well defined, and plaques rarely extend over more than four rib interspaces unless multiple and confluent. As with discrete pleural plaques, CT is more sensitive and specific for the detection of diffuse pleural thickening than chest radiography, in particular for differentiating extrapleural fat from pleural thickening. On CT, diffuse thickening appears continuous, commonly involving the posterior and lateral surfaces of the lower thorax. Frequently there is an apparent increase in extrapleural fat, partly caused by pleural retraction.

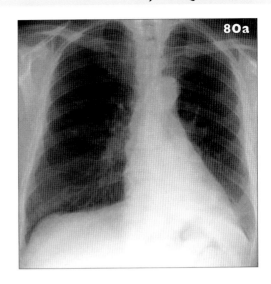

80 A 66-year-old male presented with a persistent cough and weight loss. He also reported right-sided chest pain. He had been a heavy smoker in the past but had given up 2 years previously. On examination, he was not clubbed, but had reduced air entry at the left base. He was tender over the right lower ribs in the mid axillary line. Routine blood tests were normal.

i. What does his chest radiograph show (80a)?

ii. What should be done next?

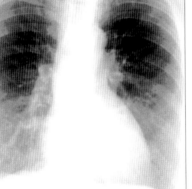

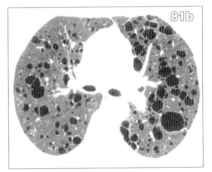

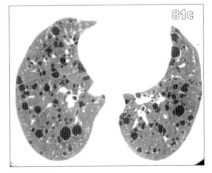

81 A 55-year-old female had presented with increasing shortness of breath. On examination, she looked well. Lung function showed a FEV$_1$ of 2.61 l (70% of predicted) and a TL$_{CO}$ 49% of predicted.

i. What do the chest radiograph (81a) and HRCT (81b, c) show?

ii. What is the likely diagnosis?

80, 81: Answers

80 i. The radiograph shows a left lower lobe collapse with increased retrocardiac density, obscuration of the left hemidiaphragm, volume loss in the left hemithorax (note the left-sided rib crowding), and depression of the left hilum (80a). There is also a subtle soft-tissue swelling related to the lateral aspect of the right 8th rib.

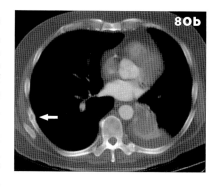

ii. The next investigations of choice would be CT and/or bronchoscopy to exclude an endobronchial lesion resulting in lobar collapse. A bronchoscopy was performed and a lesion demonstrated, which was obstructing the left lower lobe bronchus and was biopsied. Histopathology of the biopsy showed a squamous cell carcinoma.

A CT of the same case is shown imaged on bone windows (80b). The collapsed left lower lobe is demonstrated as a roughly triangular-shaped density which lies posteriorly against the thoracic spine. No air bronchograms are seen within the collapsed lobe, which is suggestive of an obstructing endobronchial lesion. The collapsed lobe is also noted to have a convex outer border which is the CT equivalent of a 'Golden's S sign' on radiography and suggests an underlying mass. There is also a small pleural effusion. The arrow shows a subtle, lucent, expansile lesion involving one of the ribs on the right which corresponds with the abnormality on the chest radiograph. These appearances are suggestive of a bony metastasis.

81 i. The chest radiograph shows hyperinflation of both lungs (81a). The HRCT demonstrates numerous thin-walled cystic airspaces uniformly distributed throughout the lungs, ranging in size from a few millimetres to 3 cm (81b, c). No other abnormality is seen in the lung parenchyma or airways.

ii. The appearances are those of lymphangioleiomyomatosis (LAM). LAM is a condition which presents in women of child-bearing age, characterized by proliferation of smooth muscle in pulmonary lymphatic vessels, blood vessels, and airways as well as the mediastinum and retroperitoneum. Patients may present with recurrent pneumothoraces, haemoptysis, and chylous pleural effusions. In this case, the history, lung function, and radiological signs are typical. Extra-pulmonary manifestations of LAM are mediastinal and abdominal angiomyolipomas.

The chest radiograph may be normal, but a nodular, reticular, or reticulonodular pattern may also be demonstrated. The lung volumes tend to increase over time, and visible cysts, bullae, or honeycomb change may develop. The HRCT appearances are of multiple thin-walled cysts which have a uniform distribution in otherwise normal lung. The cysts are often rounded with a thin wall, but may coalesce to form more bizarre shapes. The cysts are distributed throughout the lungs including the costophrenic regions, unlike the cysts in Langerhan's cell histiocytosis, which typically spare these areas, allowing radiological differentiation between the two entities.

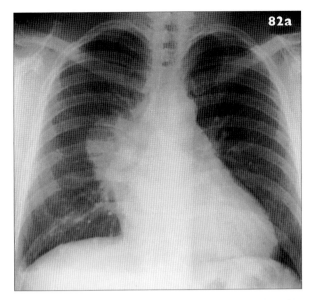

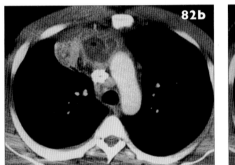

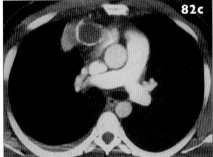

82 A 31-year-old male presented with a cough and pleuritic chest pain. He was normally fit and well and worked as an accountant. Blood tests and spirometry were normal. His chest radiograph (82a) and intravenous contrast-enhanced CT scan images (82b, c) are shown.

What is the diagnosis?

82: Answer

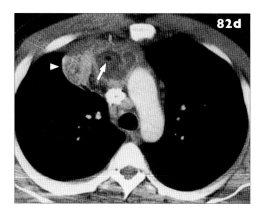

82 The chest radiograph shows abnormality of the mediastinal contour on the right with no obscuration of the right heart border or right hilum, consistent with an anterior mediastinal mass (**82a**). There is also a small right-sided pleural effusion. The contrast-enhanced CT images show the anterior mediastinal mass to be comprised of areas of differing attenuation with an area of fat (**82d**, arrow), fluid, soft tissue density, and calcification. There is some atelectasis of the adjacent anterior segment of the right upper lobe (**82d**, arrowhead). A small, right pleural effusion is confirmed on the CT. A small pretracheal lymph node is also seen at the upper limit of normal for size. The diagnosis is a benign cystic teratoma, which was confirmed by surgical resection and histopathological evaluation. The cause of the pleural effusion was presumed to be rupture into the adjacent pleural space.

Teratomas and germ cell tumours commonly arise in the mediastinum. They can be divided into benign cystic teratoma (also known as dermoid cyst) and malignant germ cell tumours such as seminomas and teratocarcinomas. Benign cystic teratomas consist primarily of ectodermal elements such as skin, hair, smooth muscle, sebaceous material, and calcification. Chest radiographic appearances are typically of a smooth well-defined or lobulated mass arising from the anterior mediastinum, often projecting to one side of the midline. Occasionally, calcification or even teeth can be visible radiographically. CT is superior to chest radiography for demonstrating areas of differing density, particularly a fatty component; demonstration of unequivocal fat or a fat–fluid level is virtually pathognomonic. Cystic components with calcified walls (as in the current case) are also common features. Rupture may occur into the adjacent lung, pleural space, or pericardium.

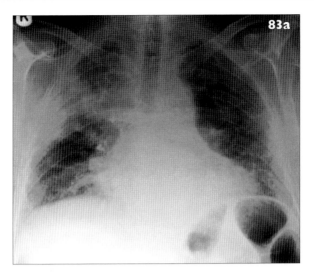

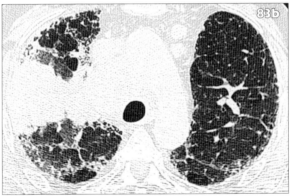

83 A 64-year-old man with known idiopathic pulmonary fibrosis (IPF) presented with weight loss and deterioration in his exercise tolerance. He had been a smoker in the past. On examination, he was apyrexial but clubbed with crackles on auscultation at both bases. His inflammatory markers were slightly raised. His pulmonary function tests showed a restrictive defect with reduction in lung volumes and transfer factor (DL_{CO}), but no recent deterioration by comparison with the last year. His chest radiograph and HRCT are shown (83a, b).

What is the likely diagnosis?

83: Answer

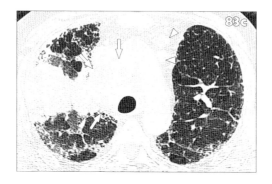

83 The chest radiograph shows features of a fibrosing lung disease with a bilateral reticular pattern and reduction in lung volume (83a). In addition, there is increased density in the right upper zone. The CT shows a bilateral reticular pattern which is most apparent in the subpleural regions, and confluent opacity in the right upper zone without air bronchograms. Despite the fact that the images are windowed for the lung, there is abnormal soft tissue visible in the right paratracheal region (83c, arrows) and a few prevascular anterior mediastinal lymph nodes to the right of the aortic arch (83c, arrowheads). While enlarged mediastinal lymph nodes (due to reactive hyperplasia) are not uncommon in IPF, the markedly enlarged right para-tracheal lymphadenopathy seems disproportionate. A bronchoscopy was performed and mucosal brushings showed a squamous cell carcinoma.

Bronchogenic carcinoma is ten to twenty times more common in patients with IPF than in the general population. Most patients with IPF have been smokers but there does seem to be a synergistic relationship between the fibrosis itself and the develop-ment of malignancy. Some series suggest that the commonest cell type is squamous cell carcinoma, followed by bronchioloalveolar cell carcinoma and adenocarcinoma. Multiple metachronous carcinomas are reported in 15% of cases. Most cancers develop in the periphery in patients with fibrosis. The radiological differential in this case would also include infection (such as tuberculosis); interestingly, community acquired pneumonias are relatively uncommon in patients with IPF.

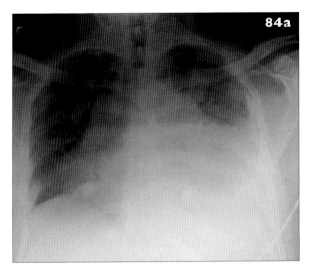

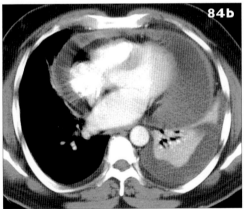

84 A 56-year-old male presented with shortness of breath and fever. He had been feeling generally unwell for a few weeks. He had been an insulin-dependent diabetic for many years, with poor attendance at the diabetic clinic. He also had a history of hypertension. He was a current smoker. He had had recent contact with his brother who had just been diagnosed with pulmonary TB and commenced on treatment. On examination he was unwell, tachycardic, and tachypnoeic. His heart sounds were quiet and the left lung base was dull to percussion. His blood glucose was slightly raised. He had an increased white cell count, and raised ESR and CRP.

What do the chest radiograph and CT show (84a, b)?

84: Answer

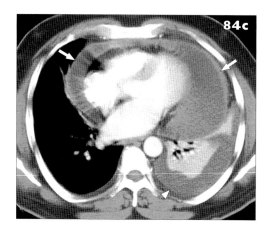

84 The chest radiograph shows an enlarged heart (despite the AP projection) which appears slightly globular in outline (84a). The left costophrenic angle appears blunted, consistent with a pleural effusion. The causes of marked cardiomegaly on radiography include ischaemic heart disease, valvular disease, cardiomyopathy, and pericardial effusion. The CT shows a left-sided pleural effusion (84c, arrowhead) with passive atelectasis of the left lower lobe. There is a rim of fluid density around the heart (84c, arrows), consistent with a large pericardial effusion. Note how the pericardium also appears thickened and shows some enhancement on the contrast-enhanced CT. The cause in this case was a tuberculous pericarditis.

There are many causes of coexisting pericardial and pleural effusions including uraemia, post-cardiac injury syndrome, tuberculosis, and malignancy. Although echocardiography is the investigation of choice for evaluating the presence of pericardial fluid, the diagnosis may be suggested from the radiograph where increasing heart size (if a series of films is available) is the most compelling sign. Pericardial fluid is easily seen on CT as a rim of fluid attenuation around the heart. The pericardial reflections extend superiorly around the ascending aorta and often pericardial fluid can be seen to extend into these recesses (particularly anteriorly in pulmonary arterial hypertension). Pericardial thickening may also be seen on CT, but a small pericardial effusion is often difficult to differentiate from pericardial thickening.

85 A 31-year-old male immigrant from the Asian subcontinent presented with a nonproductive cough and fever. On examination, he was underweight, with a fever (37.7°C; 99.9°F). His blood tests showed a raised white cell count and raised CRP. His radiograph is shown (85).
i. What is the likely diagnosis?
ii. What are the differentials for the radiographic appearances?

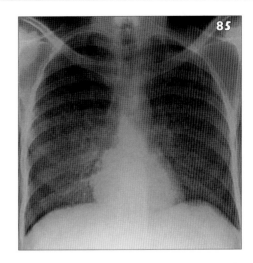

86 A 44-year-old female presented with a 2-year history of nonproductive cough and increased shortness of breath. She was a lifetime nonsmoker. She had a past history of rheumatoid arthritis and had been treated with penicillamine. She was well on examination, not clubbed or cyanosed. She had reduced breath sounds throughout both lungs. The rest of the examination was unremarkable. Lung function tests demonstrated a fixed airways obstruction with reduction of FEV_1 to 54% of predicted with a normal VC. Rheumatoid factor was positive. Bronchoscopy was normal. Open lung biopsy from the lingula and left lower lobe was performed. Inspiratory and end-expiratory CT images are shown (86a, b).
i. What are the findings?
ii. What is the probable diagnosis?

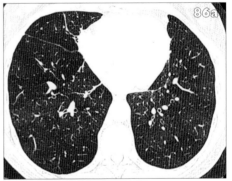

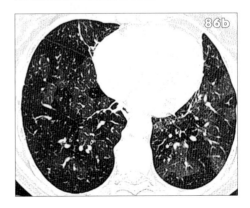

85, 86: Answers

85 i. The chest radiograph demonstrates a fine, bilateral, widespread 'miliary' nodularity (85). The cardiomediastinal contours are normal. The most likely diagnosis, given the clinical history, is miliary tuberculosis.

ii. The other radiological differentials include nontuberculous infections (e.g. histoplasmosis, coccidioidomycosis, and viral infections), miliary metastases (especially from thyroid or renal cell carcinoma, seminoma, sarcoma, or chorio-carcinoma), sarcoidosis, pneumoconioses (e.g. silicosis and coal worker's pneumo-coniosis), and alveolar microlithiasis.

Miliary tuberculosis is due to haematogenous dissemination of disease, and requires prompt diagnosis and treatment. The term 'miliary' to describe the radiographic appearances is due to the multiple, uniform, small (2–3 mm diameter) nodules which have been likened to the appearance of millet seeds.

86 i. The inspiratory HRCT shows subtle regional inhomogeneity in the density of the lung parenchyma, with areas of decreased attenuation which represent the abnormal areas (86a). The airways are minimally dilated and there is a decrease in the calibre of vessels within the blacker areas of lung. End-expiratory sections demonstrate air-trapping (a failure of the lung parenchyma to increase in attenuation on end-expiration) (86b).

ii. These findings are consistent with obliterative bronchiolitis. Histopathological findings confirmed the diagnosis and showed patchy scarring and occlusion of small airways (membranous and respiratory bronchioles). The causes of obliterative bronchiolitis include post infectious (viral), postinhalation of toxic fumes and gases (e.g. nitrogen dioxide), connective tissue disorders (such as rheumatoid arthritis), allograft recipients (bone marrow and heart–lung transplant) and drugs (such as penicillamine). In patients with rheumatoid arthritis and obliterative bronchiolitis, approximately 50% of patients have been taking penicillamine.

The chest radiograph may show hyperinflation or hypovascularity but HRCT is much more sensitive and specific. The signs on HRCT are indirect, as the small airways are themselves too small to be visualized. There is a mosaic attenuation pattern which refers to an inhomogeneity in attenuation of the lung parenchyma, the blacker areas being the abnormal areas within which there is a decrease in the calibre of vessels due to hypoxic vasoconstriction. This appearance may be relatively subtle but is accentuated on end-expiratory images, which demonstrate air-trapping. The macroscopic airways are almost invariably abnormal and appear slightly dilated and thick-walled.

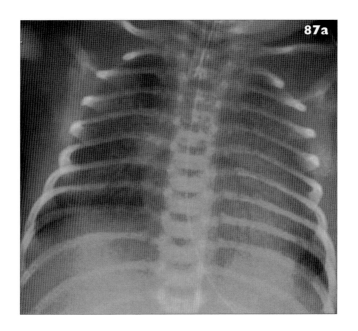

87 The chest radiograph of a neonate, born prematurely at 31 weeks' gestation, is shown (**87a**). The child developed respiratory distress shortly (24 hrs) after delivery, requiring intubation and ventilation.
i. What are the radiographic features?
ii. What is the likely cause?

87: Answer

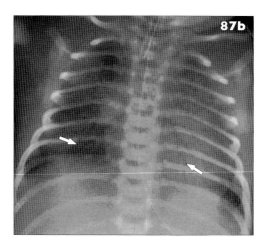

87 i. The radiograph shows an endotracheal tube and nasogastric tube in place. There is bilateral airspace opacity throughout the lungs with air bronchograms (**87b,** arrows) seen as branching linear lucencies within areas of consolidation.

ii. The likely cause is respiratory distress syndrome (RDS) (hyaline membrane disease). RDS is the commonest life-threatening respiratory condition in neonates. It usually occurs in premature neonates due to surfactant deficiency or ineffectiveness. The role of surfactant (a phospholipid secreted by Type II pneumocytes) is the prevention of alveolar collapse by decreasing surface tension as lung volume decreases. If surfactant is deficient or ineffective, an adhesive atelectasis occurs. Approximately 50% of neonates born between 26 and 28 weeks' gestation and 20–30% born at 30–31 weeks' gestation develop RDS. The condition is unusual after 36 weeks' gestation, where other risk factors such as poorly controlled maternal diabetes and multiple gestations play a role. In recent years, pre-natal stimulation of surfactant production with corticosteriods and post-natal use of synthetic or natural surfactants have had an impact on prevention and reduction of severity of the disease.

The chest radiograph is usually abnormal within 6 hours after birth, showing decreased aeration of the lungs, as opposed to the increased aeration seen in transient tachypnoea of the newborn. Initially in RDS, there is a fine reticular pattern with air bronchograms throughout both lungs due to the terminal airways being surrounded by airless alveoli. With progressive disease, the reticulonodular shadowing becomes symmetrically more confluent and there is obscuration of the diaphragmatic and mediastinal contours.

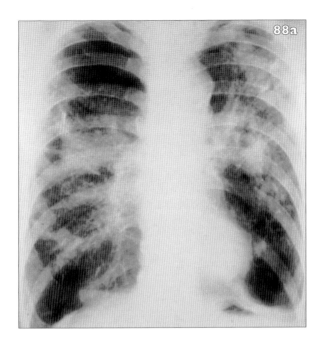

88 An 82-year-old male presented with increasing breathlessness on exertion, which had progressed over 1 year. His symptoms had started at the age of 64, necessitating retirement from coal mining. He also complained of a nonproductive cough and right-sided pleuritic chest pain. He had a 40-pack-year smoking history but had recently stopped smoking. His past medical history included an episode of pneumonia 10 years previously. He was not breathless at rest and was not cyanosed or clubbed. Chest expansion was decreased on the right and bronchial breathing and coarse crepitations were heard on auscultation at the right base. Full blood count and urea and electrolytes were normal. He was mildly hypoxic on room air (pO$_2$: 79 mmHg; 10.53 kPa). A bronchoscopy was normal, apart from demonstrating coal deposits in the large airways. A bronchoalveolar lavage was performed, but cytology showed no malignant cells.

What is the diagnosis from the chest radiograph (88a)?

88: Answer

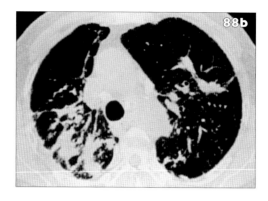

88 The chest radiograph shows multiple bilateral large mid-zone opacities on a background of fine nodularity (88a). There is bilateral upper-zone volume loss and both hila are displaced superiorly. There are calcified mediastinal lymph nodes. An HRCT examination shows large asymmetrical irregular opacities of varying sizes with parenchymal distortion in the upper lobes bilaterally (88b). Some opacities are calcified. There are also diffuse, small, well-defined 2–3 mm nodules throughout the lungs, some of which are subpleural. The calcified mediastinal lymph nodes are also demonstrated.

The radiological appearances are those of coal worker's pneumoconiosis complicated by progressive massive fibrosis and are images of the same individual in Question 16, taken 16 years later. Another possible cause, in the absence of an occupational history, would have been pulmonary sarcoidosis. The radiographic appearances of coal worker's pneumoconiosis and silicosis are similar: both conditions are characterized by a predominance of upper-zone nodules which have the propensity to coalesce to form conglomerate masses (progressive massive fibrosis). Progressive massive fibrosis (PMF) manifests as mass-like opacities, usually in the posterior upper lobes with hilar retraction. Over a period of time, the masses may appear to migrate towards the hila. The masses are usually symmetric but can be unilateral. The presence of coexisting lobar volume loss and peripheral cicatricial emphysema may be helpful in differentiating unilateral PMF from lung cancer. On CT, PMF appears as irregular upper-lobe masses which are often bilateral and calcified, with a background of centrilobular nodules. There may be paracicatricial emphysema and thickening of adjacent extrapleural fat.

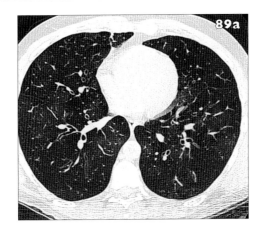

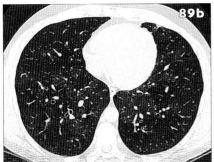
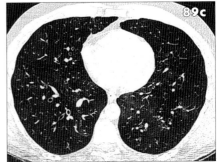

89 An HRCT is shown of a 43-year-old male who underwent an allogeneic (from a donor) bone marrow transplant for chronic myeloid leukaemia 18 months previously. His chest radiograph (not shown) was normal. He became increasingly more short of breath, with an obstructive defect on pulmonary function testing. The HRCT is shown with images in inspiration (89a, b) and end-expiration (89c).

What complication has occurred?

89: Answer

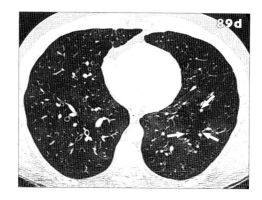

89 The HRCTs show abnormality of the large airways, which are mildly bronchiectatic by HRCT criteria. There is a mosaic attenuation pattern which is accentuated on the end-expiratory image, indicating areas of air-trapping (89d, arrows). The appearances are those of obliterative bronchiolitis due to graft-versus-host disease affecting the lungs.

Chronic graft-versus-host disease is a manifestation of organ transplantation seen in allogeneic bone marrow transplants, heart–lung transplants and single or double lung transplantation. Autologous bone marrow transplants (where the patient's own bone marrow is harvested) are not usually associated with graft-versus-host disease and obliterative bronchiolitis has only rarely been reported. Chronic graft-versus-host disease is a late complication, occurring after 3 months following organ transplantation, and is characterized histopathologically by an obliterative bronchiolitis and lymphocytic airway infiltration. The radiographic features are often subtle and nonspecific and the radiograph may be normal initially. Airway dilatation and thickening with hyperinflation (representing air-trapping) may be seen. HRCT features include bronchiectasis (which may be more subtle than in this case) and a mosaic attenuation pattern which is accentuated on end-expiratory images with evidence of air-trapping. The diagnosis is often confirmed histopathologically as the condition may be reversible with appropriate modification of immunosuppressant therapy.

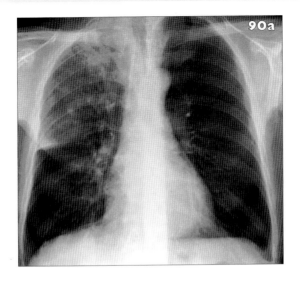

90 A previously fit and healthy 37-year-old male presented with a productive cough and fever. His symptoms had been present for 1 week. He was a nonsmoker with no pets and no recent travel abroad. There were no risk factors for HIV infection. On examination, he was tachycardic and pyrexial, but not clubbed. He had a raised white cell count (neutrophilia), CRP and ESR. His radiograph is shown (**90a**).

What is the radiographic differential diagnosis?

91 A 24-year-old male presented with lethargy and feeling unwell. He was normally fit and well and an active sportsman. There were no abnormalities to find on examination. His full blood count and urea and electrolytes were normal. His chest radiograph is shown (**91**).
i. What are the findings?
ii. Suggest a possible diagnosis.

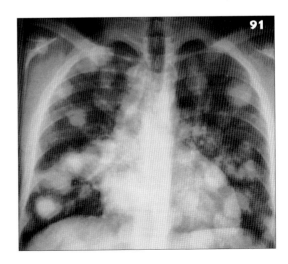

90, 91: Answers

90 The radiograph shows consolidation within the right upper lobe. The consolidation is bounded inferiorly by the horizontal fissure, but there is no volume loss. There are air bronchograms within the consolidation (90b, arrows). The radiographic appearances are of lobar pneumonia.

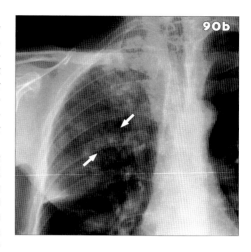

The commonest cause of a lobar consolidation is a community-acquired pneumonia. An inflammatory exudate begins peripherally in the airspaces and spreads across segments via the pores of Kohn, resulting in homogeneous consolidation (usually with air bronchograms). There is no associated volume loss and the affected lobe may occasionally be expanded. Consolidation is often confined to a single lobe and multilobar disease is relatively uncommon in a straightforward community-acquired pneumonia. Common organisms include *Streptococcus pneumoniae*, *S. pyogenes*, and *Staphylococcus aureus*. *S. pneumoniae* (pneumococcal) pneumonia is the commonest community-acquired pneumonia and may occur at any age. Predisposing factors include previous splenectomy and various chronic diseases. Infection with *Mycobacterium tuberculosis* should also be considered.

91 i. The chest radiograph shows multiple, large (2–3 cm diameter) well-defined nodules in both lungs (91).
ii. The differential diagnosis includes metastastic disease (most commonly from breast, thyroid, gastrointestinal tract, and testicular malignancies), widespread abscesses (although cavitation would be expected), Wegener's granulomatosis, rheumatoid nodules, and rare infections such as hydatid. The diagnosis of multiple metastases from a testicular germ cell tumour was made.

The prevalence of pulmonary metastases depends on the stage of disease and the primary tumour. Although tumours such as choriocarcinoma, osteosarcoma, melanoma, and thyroid carcinoma are frequently associated with pulmonary metastases, other malignancies (breast, colon, kidney, uterus) and head and neck tumours are commoner in the general population and thus these are the commonest primaries found in patients with disseminated disease in autopsy series. The usual appearance of haematogenous pulmonary metastases is multiple, well-defined, rounded lesions throughout the lungs, more frequent in the outer and lower zones. The size varies from a few millimetres to several centimetres, as in this case.

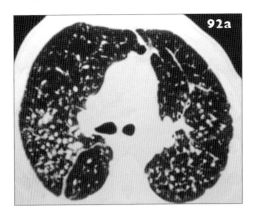

92 A 59-year-old male presented with cough and increasing shortness of breath on exertion. He had worked for many years in a light bulb factory and was a nonsmoker. On examination, he was not clubbed or short of breath at rest. His chest radiograph (not shown) demonstrated a bilateral reticulonodular pattern affecting the mid and upper zones. There was the impression of hilar lymphadenopathy.

i. What does the HRCT show (92a)?
ii. What is the likely diagnosis?

93 A 75-year-old male's radiograph is shown (93). He had been treated for tuberculosis (TB) many years previously.

What treatment had been performed?

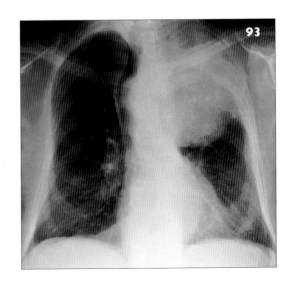

92, 93: Answers

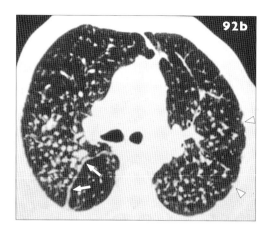

92 i. The HRCT shows a nodular pattern. There is a subpleural predominance with nodules seen along the fissure (92b, arrowheads) and in the peripheral subpleural areas of the lung (92b, arrows). Mediastinal windows show mediastinal and hilar lymphadenopathy.

ii. The CT appearances are those of sarcoidosis or, with this occupational history, berylliosis.

Berylliosis is less common nowadays due to recognition of the toxic effects of the element. Beryllium was used in the fluorescent-light industry, but is also now encountered in the aerospace, ceramics, and nuclear power industries. Histopathologically, the condition is characterized by the presence of noncaseating granulomas and, in the chronic form, is indistinguishable histopathologically and radiologically from pulmonary sarcoidosis. Acute berylliosis may result from a single intense exposure and presents as acute tracheobronchitis and pulmonary oedema.

The radiographic appearances of chronic berylliosis include hilar and mediastinal lymphadenopathy, and a bilateral reticulonodular pattern without any particular zonal predominance. As the disease progresses, there may be volume loss and fibrosis and enlargement of the central pulmonary arteries reflecting pulmonary arterial hypertension. The HRCT features are indistinguishable from those of pulmonary sarcoidosis.

93 The radiograph shows the appearances of plombage, which involved the instillation of inert material (e.g. paraffin, adipose tissue, lucite spheres, or plastic) into the pleural space as a treatment for TB (93). It was used in place of thoracoplasty as it was less deforming for the patient and lung function was preserved. The practice is very uncommon nowadays but was prevalent in the middle of the twentieth century. Complications include extrusion of plombage material outside the pleural space, bronchopleural fistula and, rarely, the development of carcinoma or sarcoma.

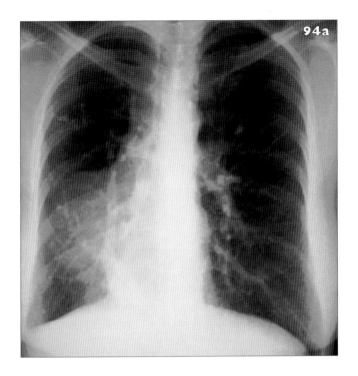

94 The chest radiograph of a 20-year-old female who had been treated for a ventriculoseptal defect as a child is shown (**94a**). Since her surgery she had been well, with no complaints and had worked as a secretary. She was a nonsmoker and was not taking any medication.

What congenital abnormality is shown?

94: Answer

94 The radiograph shows the right lung to be small, with right-sided volume loss and increased opacification in the right lower zone (**94a**). A tubular structure is seen to course vertically within the right lower zone medially to the right hemidiaphragm. The right hilum is abnormally small and it is difficult to identify the right pulmonary artery. There is dextropositioning of the heart. The appearances are of a scimitar syndrome (hypogenetic lung syndrome or congenital pulmonary venolobar syndrome).

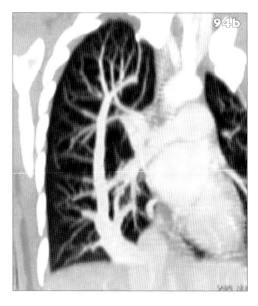

The condition almost always occurs within the right lung which is hypoplastic with underdevelopment of the bronchial tree and vascular structures. There is often a reduction in the number and size of bronchi and the pulmonary artery is small, with abnormal systemic arterial supply to the underlying lung. The syndrome is named after the anomalous draining vein which is often seen as a vertical curvilinear structure on the radiograph, resembling a Turkish sword or scimitar. The abnormal vein may drain the whole lung or only part directly through the diaphragm into the inferior vena cava.

Approximately one-quarter of cases are associated with congenital cardiac anomalies, the commonest being septal defects. In cases uncomplicated by cardiac defects, the syndrome is compatible with normal life expectancy. Other associated abnormalities include Bochdalek hernias, tracheal diverticula, bronchiectasis, and horseshoe kidney. Although the draining vein is often well demonstrated on the radiograph, either CT or MR shows the venous anatomy to superior effect with multiplanar imaging capabilities (**94b**). CT may be useful in demonstrating associated airway abnormalities and horseshoe lung.

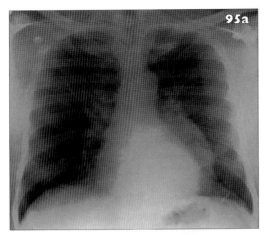
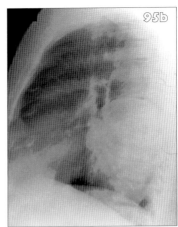
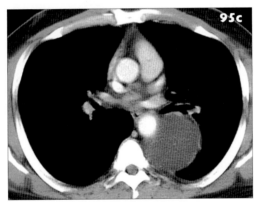

95 A 29-year-old male presented to his family doctor with a cough productive of sputum for several weeks. Initial treatment with a course of antibiotics did not alleviate his symptoms and he was referred for a chest radiograph. He had no previous medical history and had been well. He was a nonsmoker and worked in information technology. On examination, there were no abnormalites to find. His frontal and lateral radiographs (95a, b) are shown with an intravenous contrast-enhanced CT (95c).

What are the possible diagnoses?

95: Answer

95 The frontal and lateral chest radiographs show a large posterior mediastinal mass (95a, b). The CT shows the mass to lie to the left of the aorta, with no contrast enhancement and low attenuation suggestive of fluid density (95c). The differential for mediastinal fluid-filled structures includes bronchogenic cysts, oesophageal duplication cysts, neurenteric cysts, pericardial cysts, thymic cysts, pancreatic pseudocysts, cystic hygromas, and lymphoceles (post-traumatic). Due to the position of the cyst, the differential of a bronchogenic cyst, oesophageal duplication cyst, and neurenteric cyst is most likely. MRI was performed to determine whether there were any associated vertebral body abnormalities or a communication with the subarachnoid space to suggest a neurenteric cyst, but none were demonstrated (95d). The MRI showed communication with the oesophagus, consistent with an oesophageal duplication cyst.

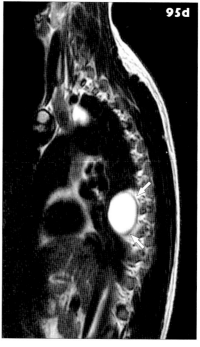

Oesophageal duplication cysts may present in children or adults. Most are asymptomatic and are often discovered incidentally on imaging for other reasons. However, there may be pressure effects if the cyst is large and dysphagia and pain may be presenting features. The imaging features are very similar to those of a bronchogenic cyst, although the lesion may be tubular and sometimes thick-walled and in close contact with the oesophagus (giving a clue as to its origin). On MRI, the cyst may be high signal on both T1- and T2-weighted images, reflecting the proteinaceous nature of the fluid (arrows).

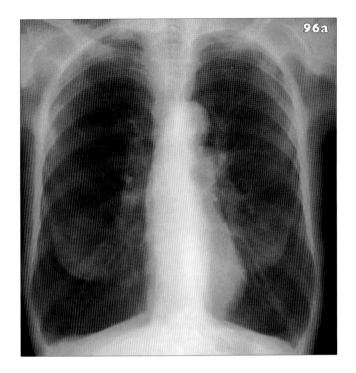

96 A 63- year-old female had been complaining of increasing shortness of breath and weight loss over several years. Her exercise tolerance had diminished and she had become dyspnoeic on minimal extertion. She was a heavy smoker (40 pack-years). On examination, she was clubbed, very thin, and slightly tachypnoeic. She was noted to be using her accessory muscles of respiration at rest. On percussion her chest was hyper-resonant with diminished breath sounds. Her lung function tests showed an obstructive defect with a marked reduction in K_{CO} (42% of predicted).

i. What does the chest radiograph (96a) show and what is the likely diagnosis?
ii. What might you expect to see on CT?

96: Answer

96 i. The chest radiograph shows both hemidiaphragms to be low and flattened (**96a**). The combination of diaphragmatic flattening and depression is a relatively specific radiographic feature of emphysema, whereas depression alone may be seen in overinflation in conditions such as asthma. Normally, in the midclavicular line, the right hemidiaphragm should be above the anterior end of the seventh rib. Flattening of the diaphragm can be assessed by joining a line between the costophrenic and cardio-phrenic angles and, if the maximum per-pendicular height from this line to the edge of the diaphragm is <1.5 cm, flattening is present. On a lateral radiograph the retro-sternal airspace may be enlarged. The lungs may be generally or focally of increased transradiancy, with a reduction in the size and number of vascular markings with

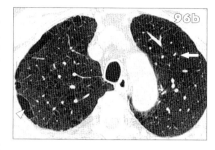

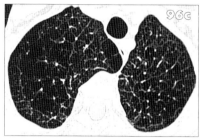

vascular distortion. However, the vascular features of emphysema may be more subjective than diaphragmatic flattening and are associated with high interobserver variation.

Despite the specificity of diaphragmatic flattening and depression, radiography is relatively insensitive for detection of mild or moderate emphysema. By contrast, HRCT is very sensitive and the features that are described in early centrilobular emphysema are areas of permeative destruction or decreased attenuation without definable walls in the centre of the secondary pulmonary lobule, adjacent to the artery (**96b**, arrow). As the emphysema becomes more extensive, the areas of parenchymal destruction may have definable walls as they are bounded by interlobular septa as seen in **96c**. Other features include bullae (focal cysts with well-defined, very thin walls), vascular distortion, and pruning and attenuation of vessels.

ii. CT can also differentiate between the different types of emphysema. Centrilobular emphysema is the commonest type associated with cigarette smoking and tends to have an upper-lobe predilection initially. With severe disease it becomes more widespread, but typically remains most severe in the upper lobes. Paraseptal emphysema is often considered as part of centrilobular emphysema, and is also associated with cigarette smoking. The distribution of destruction is peripherally within the secondary pulmonary lobule, and cystic airspaces with visible 'hairline' walls are seen along the interlobular septa (thus paraseptal emphysema) and in a subpleural distribution (**96b**, arrowhead). Panacinar emphysema is seen in alpha-1-antitrypsin deficiency (see Question **13**).

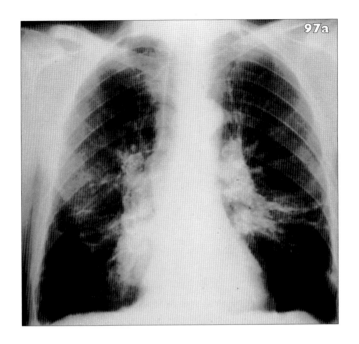

97 The radiograph of a 56-year-old male is shown who had worked for several years as a sandblaster (**97a**). He was mildly dyspnoeic on exertion and had also been a heavy smoker in the past.
i. What are the radiological findings?
ii. What is the likely diagnosis?

97: Answer

97 i. The radiograph shows bilateral hilar enlargement with a lobulated outline and 'egg-shell' or peripheral calcification (97b, arrows). Subtle small nodules are seen within both upper and mid zones and the lungs are of large volume with flattening of the hemi-diaphragms, suggestive of obstructive lung disease.

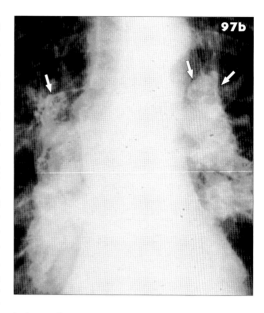

ii. The appearances are typical of silicosis with coexisting emphysema. The incidence of silicosis has fallen in recent years. Quarry workers, sandblasters, and masonry cutters and polishers are susceptible, as silicon dioxide is present in many rocks in the Earth's crust, particularly quartz. Acute silicoproteinosis occurs after heavy exposure in confined spaces, and radiologically resembles alveolar proteinosis (see Question 36). In the chronic form of the disease, radiographic findings are very similar to those of simple coal worker's pneumoconiosis (see Question 16), with small, well-defined, upper- and mid-zone nodules which may be calcified. Mediastinal and hilar lymphadenopathy are common, and the nodes are often calcified peripherally, resulting in so-called 'egg-shell' calcification. The HRCT appearances are also similar to those of simple coal worker's pneumoconiosis, with small subpleural and centrilobular nodules. Progressive massive fibrosis may also develop with nodules >1 cm in diameter, which gradually migrate towards the hila over time. Although a large proportion of individuals with simple silicosis or coal worker's pneumoconiosis are current or ex-smokers and have coexisting emphysema, emphysema is also a feature in cases where there is no smoking history. The small nodules in simple silicosis and coal worker's pneumoconiosis are not usually associated with a functional defect; however, co-existing emphysema may result in dyspnoea and an obstructive defect on lung function testing.

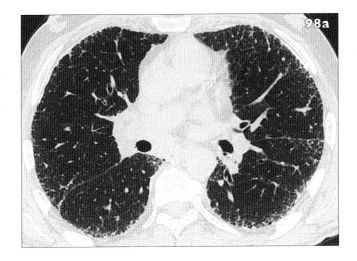

98 A former shipyard worker presented with a gradual history of increasing shortness of breath on exertion. He had been a shipfitter for 20 years and had had a clerical job for the next 15 years. On examination, he was slightly short of breath at rest and clubbed. On auscultation, fine inspiratory crackles were heard. On lung function testing, he had a restrictive defect with a reduction in lung volumes and gas transfer (DL_{CO}). The chest radiograph is not shown. An HRCT was performed (98a).
i. What are the HRCT features?
ii. What is the likely diagnosis?
iii. What is the next test to be performed?

98: Answer

98 i. The HRCT shows a fine, subpleural reticular pattern. There are calcified pleural plaques under the anterior ends of the ribs which are more apparent on the soft tissue windows (98b, arrows).

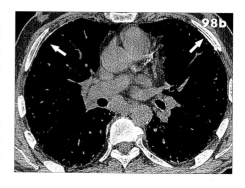

ii. The diagnosis of interstitial pulmonary fibrosis due to asbestos exposure (asbestosis) was made on a combination of the history of the exposure intensity and duration, in addition to the clinical, pulmonary function, and radiological findings.

iii. Further tests are not usually required and an open lung biopsy in cases of suspected asbestosis is not recommended by most authorities (including the American Thoracic Society). Histopathologically, asbestos or ferruginous bodies are not specific for the diagnosis of asbestosis and may occur in individuals who have been environmentally, rather than occupationally exposed.

Asbestosis usually occurs many (20–30) years after exposure and a reliable history of nontrivial exposure is mandatory for the diagnosis. Crocidolite is the most fibrogenic form. Histopathologically, early disease is characterized by a peribronchiolar distribution of fibrosis, which is often apparent in the subpleural regions of the lung, but as the disease progresses distinction from idiopathic pulmonary fibrosis becomes more difficult. The radiographic features may be identical to those of idiopathic pulmonary fibrosis (IPF), apart from the presence of pleural disease such as pleural plaques and diffuse pleural thickening. Initial features include basal groundglass and reticular opacities which may progress to involve the whole lung, including the upper lobes, with volume loss and honeycombing. The HRCT parenchymal features are also often identical to those of IPF, with a basal, subpleural reticular pattern or honeycombing. In very early disease, the peribronchiolar distribution of fibrosis in asbestosis may be apparent as subpleural dots which can help differentiate it from IPF but, depending on the type of exposure, asbestos-induced disease is often more advanced at presentation. There is controversy over whether parenchymal bands radiating from areas of pleural thickening into the lung parenchyma represent true 'asbestosis' or parenchymal changes as a result of pleural thickening. Most authorities favour the latter explanation and suggest that these areas may represent early folded lung or rounded atelectasis (see Question 79).

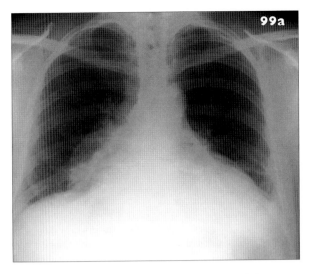

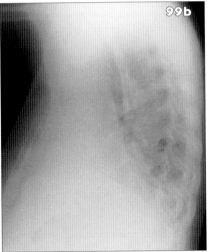

99 A normally fit and well 36-year-old male presented with a cough and feeling generally unwell to his family doctor. He was a nonsmoker and normally worked as a security guard. On examination, he was well with no abnormal findings in his respiratory or cardiovascular systems. A chest radiograph was requested as his symptoms had not responded to a course of antibiotics.

i. What does the chest radiograph (PA and right lateral, **99a, b**) show?

ii. What examination should be performed next?

99: Answer

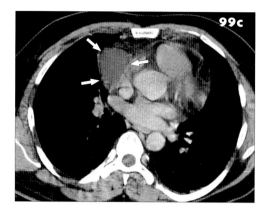

99 i. The PA and right lateral radiographs show abnormal density within the anterior mediastinum, adjacent to the right heart border (99a, b). Note how the right hilar structures are not obscured on the frontal radiograph. The obscuration of the outline of the left hemidiaphragm is likely to be due to the patient's suboptimal inspiratory effort. The differential diagnosis includes causes of anterior mediastinal masses (see Question 32). Another diagnosis to consider would be a pericardial cyst because of the relationship to the right heart border.

ii. A CT was performed next. The abnormality is shown to be adjacent to the right atrium (99c, arrows) and of fluid attenuation. The diagnosis of a pericardial cyst was made and the abnormality spontaneously regressed on subsequent radiographs.

Pericardial cysts arise owing to anomalous outpouchings of the parietal pericardium. They are often asymptomatic and discovered incidentally; however, patients may present with chest pain, cough, and shortness of breath. If aspirated, clear yellow fluid is the typical finding, and cysts are more often unilocular than multilocular. Histopathologically, the wall is composed of collagen lined by a single layer of mesothelial cells.

The cysts are commoner on the right than the left and usually occur in the anterior cardiophrenic regions, directly contacting adjacent structures such as the heart, diaphragm, and chest wall. The cysts are seen as smooth, well-defined rounded structures on radiography and CT, contacting the cardiac borders. Calcification is unusual and the fluid density is readily demonstrated with CT, although ultrasound or MRI may also confirm the findings.

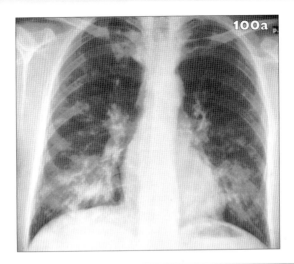

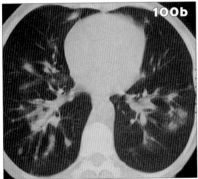

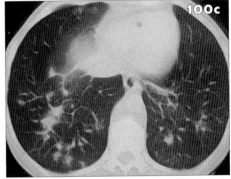

100 A 35-year-old male was diagnosed as HIV-positive, as well as having positive hepatitis A and C serology at presentation. Five years later he developed oral candidiasis. Subsequently he was diagnosed as having multi-focal cutaneous Kaposi's sarcoma, which responded to antiretroviral agents. He presented a further 2 years later with a 4-week history of haemoptysis and weight loss. On examination, he was apyrexial with an oxygen saturation of 98%, and no significant desaturation on exercise. Oral candidiasis was noted. Auscultation of his chest was unremarkable. The CD4 lymphocyte count was 2×10^9/l (2000/mm³) (normal range 0.7–1.35 $\times 10^9$/l [700–1350/mm³]). Sputum cultures were negative. Bronchoscopy was normal, and bronchoalveolar lavage was negative for acid-fast bacilli and *Pneumocystis carinii*.

i. What do the chest radiograph (100a) and HRCT (100b, c) show?
ii. Give the likely diagnosis.

100: Answer

100 i. The chest radiograph shows a perihilar infiltrate with peribronchial thickening (100a). There are numerous soft tissue nodules, predominantly in the mid zones and more confluent shadowing at the bases. The HRCT scans demonstrate broncho-vascular thickening and multiple spiculated nodules of varying sizes, concentrated mainly around the bronchovascular bundles (100b, c). Small lymph nodes were found to be present in the pretracheal, subcarinal, and para-aortic regions (not shown). There are also a few thickened interlobular septa at the lung bases.

ii. A diagnosis of pulmonary Kaposi's sarcoma (KS) was made on the basis of the clinical and radiological findings. KS is the most common AIDS-related malignant disease, affecting 25% of AIDS patients, and occurs mainly in homosexual or bisexual men. This trend is due to an infectious aetiology, with human herpes virus-8 having been cited as the most likely causative agent. Pulmonary involvement occurs in up to 50% of patients with cutaneous KS; only occasionally does pulmonary KS occur before a diagnosis of cutaneous disease has been established. It more commonly afflicts patients with a low CD4 count. Typical radiographic findings include thickening along the bronchovascular bundles spreading peripherally from a perihilar origin, reflecting the propensity of KS to grow in the peribronchial and perivascular axial interstitial spaces. These result in characteristic 'flame-shaped' opacities. Later nodular change occurs, which may coalesce to dense confluent opacities. The mid and lower zones are most frequently affected. Interlobular septal thickening, pleural effusions, endobronchial lesions, and mediastinal lymphadenopathy are also relatively common findings.

Further reading and useful websites

American Journal of Roentgenology (http://www.ajronline.org/)

Clinical Radiology (http://www.harcourt-international.com/journals/crad/)

European Society of Thoracic Imaging (http://www.esti-society.org/)

Fraser and Pare's Diagnosis of Diseases of the Chest. Richard S Fraser, PD Pare. WB Saunders.

Grainger and Allison's Diagnostic Radiology: A Textbook of Medical Imaging. Ronald G Grainger, David J Allison, Andreas Adam (Editor), Adrian K. Dixon (Editor). Churchill Livingstone (2001).

High Resolution CT of the Lungs (3rd edn) W Richard Webb, Nestor L Muller, David P Naidich. Lippincott Williams and Wilkins (2000).

Imaging of Diseases of the Chest. David M Hansell, Peter Armstrong, David A Lynch, H Page McAdams. Mosby (2004).

Principles of Chest Roentgenology: A Programmed Text (2nd edn). Benjamin Felson, Lawrence R Goodman (editor). Saunders (1999)

Radiology (http://radiology.rsnajnls.org/)

Society of Thoracic Imaging (http://www.thoracicrad.org/str2000/)

Index

Index

Index